THE CHILD
IN MIND

A CHILD PROTECTION HANDBOOK
Revised edition

Judy Barker and Deborah T. Hodes

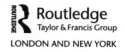

Routledge
Taylor & Francis Group

LONDON AND NEW YORK

First published in 2002 by City and Hackney Primary Care Trust

This revised edition published 2004
by Routledge
2 Park Square, Milton Park, Abingdon, Oxon, OX14 4RN

Simultaneously published in the USA and Canada
by Routledge
270 Madison Ave, New York, NY 10016

Routledge is an imprint of the Taylor & Francis Group, an informa business

© 2004 Judy Barker and Deborah T. Hodes

Reprinted 2005, 2006

The right of Judy Barker and Deborah T. Hodes to be identified as the Authors of this Work has been asserted by them in accordance with the Copyright, Designs and Patents Act 1988

Typeset in Frutiger by Taylor & Francis Books Ltd

Printed and bound in Great Britain by TJ International Ltd, Padstow, Cornwall

British Library Cataloguing in Publication Data
A catalogue record for this book is available from the British Library

Library of Congress Cataloging in Publication Data
A catalog record for this book has been requested

ISBN10 0–415–32174–3 (hbk)
ISBN10 0–415–32175–1 (pbk)
ISBN13 978–0–415–32174–7 (hbk)
ISBN13 978–0–415–32175–4 (pbk)

To our parents
and our children Clara, Daniel, Emilio, Lydia and Matthew

Contents

FOREWORD
by Claire Rayner

There are several different points of view about the incidence of child abuse in this country at this time.

There is the all too common response that abuse is the direct result of the unique wickedness of our modern society, the death of deference and God-fearing good behaviour. People who take this view find it hard to be convinced, even when presented with documentary evidence, that child abuse existed and may even have been worse in the so-called 'Good Old Days'.

Then there are those who see the incidence of this distressing problem of modern society as entirely the result of political ineptitude. For them, it is the State's failure to provide for the poorest members of society, dooming them to inadequate housing in depressing milieux, providing minimal standards of care for those unable to earn adequate living wages for themselves, and only the most basic of educational opportunities for the children of the uneducated, that is at the root of the problem. These people need to be convinced that child abuse is not behaviour limited only to the poor and uneducated, but is just as likely to occur in middle- and even upper-class circles.

This confusion of ideas about child abuse is not confined to the general public. Every professional working with children and their families, be they doctors or teachers, nurses or dentists, and every person working alongside them in an administrative or clerical capacity, is part of the general public and will not necessarily have had the opportunity to find out the facts about child abuse for themselves.

And that is why this book is so important. It offers in clear direct prose (blessedly free of jargon, glory be!) all that we need to know about the forms of abuse a child may suffer, how they may be recognised and how they should be dealt with, taking care to cause the least possible damage to an already damaged child.

It is also blessedly free of any of the hysteria that appears, notably in the popular press but also in society as a whole, whenever cases of child abuse are discovered. If you listen to people in shops, offices or pubs discussing issues around widely publicised cases of child abuse, the degree of ignorance displayed is depressing indeed. And we must not forget that well over three-quarters of the population consider it perfectly proper to use corporal punishment on small children and fail totally to see any connection between such actions and the child abuse they discuss.

This is a book that should be in everyone's back pocket, but most particularly in those of every health worker, so that it is available at all times for rapid consultation. It has been designed to fit into the national strategy for child protection, but even without that link, it is an excellent tool for anyone who truly cares about, and wishes to do the best for, children and families. It is a pleasure to recommend it so heartily.

Acknowledgements

We should like to thank Sue Dutch and Laura Sharpe for supporting the initial publication and Helen Armitage for her skilful editing. We thank Elaine Merrin, Chris Hobbs, Danya Glaser, Jane Watkeys, Debbie Xavier and Vic Larcher for kindly reading through the manuscript and making many helpful suggestions.

The acknowledged inspiration for the title of this handbook is *A Child In Mind: Protection of Children in a Responsible Society*, the report of the Commission of Inquiry into the circumstances surrounding the death of Kimberley Carlile, first published by the London Borough of Greenwich in 1987.

Appendix 1: The Assessment Framework is reproduced from *Working Together to Safeguard Children*. (DH, 1999)

Introduction

Whether a nurse, doctor, dentist or allied health professional, manager or administrative or clerical worker, the contribution of all health service workers to the protection of children is crucial. The welfare of children and in some cases a child's life depends not only on professional vigilance and a willingness to consider the possibility of child abuse and neglect but also on action taken in response to it. It depends on asking the child, listening to what they say; sometimes believing things people think do not, could not or should not happen to children.

The inquiry into the death of Victoria Climbié from abuse and neglect found the professional network failed to act on concerns about her safety and welfare. It said that there were many occasions when intervention could have saved her life. All these opportunities were lost, not because nobody suspected she was being abused but because nobody followed the most straightforward procedures in response to suspicions that she was being deliberately harmed.

Ensuring the safety and promoting the welfare of children who are at risk of harm is not an easy undertaking. It is sometimes difficult to assess the significance of the information about a child, to gauge its seriousness or decide what to do next. It is easy to lose a sense of perspective and the focus on the child in an attempt also to take into account the needs of the parent/carer, family and professional network. In acknowledging this *The Child in Mind* is a guide to how to keep the focus on the child: how to keep the child in mind. Its practical approach aims to inform professional judgements about how best to protect the child within the context of their family and wider environment.

It is not necessary to be an expert in paediatrics or child abuse to have concerns about a child but following child-protection guidelines once abuse is suspected is a requirement for everyone, managers and clinicians alike. *The Child in Mind* recognises that child protection is a responsibility which crosses all services and all hierarchies. It places equal value on each person's contribution to the process of protecting

children, and its guidance is designed to inform everyone working in the
health service as well as workers in other agencies. None of the material
is exclusive to any one agency or individual worker; for example, the
reader may choose the degree of detail they feel they require in order
best to understand physical or child sexual abuse. Those working
alongside doctors and who refer children to them may find information
about the paediatric assessment helpful to an understanding of what
doctors do and how they contribute to the child protection process.

The Child in Mind provides a context for the local Area Child
Protection Committee (ACPC) procedures and the national framework
for child protection practice, *Working Together to Safeguard Children*,
and is designed to be used in conjunction with them and, indeed, other
more detailed textbooks, reports and journals. Furthermore, it is
intended to complement the arrangements for consultation, supervision
and training that already exist in every health service trust.

1

Safeguarding children

It is estimated that between 2 and 4 children die every week as a consequence of abuse and/or neglect and many more suffer irreversible long-term effects. Nearly all these children will come into contact with a health professional at some point in their lives. A large proportion of child protection referrals are made by health service staff, and many of the services that make a difference to the quality of life for these children are provided by professionals working in a variety of disciplines within the health service. All these practitioners have information that may prove significant for children at risk.

Health care workers have a distinct contribution to make to the protection of children – from prevention of abuse to its identification, through monitoring the health and development of children who have been abused, to therapeutic intervention and the prevention of further abuse. Their role in the care of children and families is key not only to preventing abuse but also to safeguarding vulnerable children once abuse has started.

Health service staff working in all fields may at some time come into contact with children who are at risk of abuse and/or neglect; for example those involved in adult-focused services, such as mental health or drug and alcohol services, will be in contact with adults whose problems may adversely affect children in their care. Child protection is therefore integral to the provision of any health service. While some practitioners offer advice to families on how to promote health and prevent illness and disability, others deal with acutely ill children and families in crisis. Wherever they are working, health care workers are key to the prevention of child maltreatment and the early identification of abuse and neglect.

Working together to safeguard children

Working Together to Safeguard Children (DH, 1999) is the national framework for child protection practice and its guidance applies to everyone working with children and families. It explains how the child protection process works, setting out the responsibilities of professionals and the procedures to follow when there are concerns about a child. One of the principles of *Working Together* and the accompanying *Framework for the Assessment of Children in Need and Their Families* (DH, 2000) is that child protection practice should operate within a broader framework of children in need. This includes the needs of children who are, for example, looked-after, disabled, abused through prostitution or suffer social exclusion. These two documents set out the national strategy for children in need and children in need of protection; they also stress the particular importance of an integrated multi-professional approach by all agencies to the assessment and planning processes for all vulnerable children.

What To Do If You're Worried a Child is Being Abused (DH, 2003) is a short guide written in response to the issues raised in the Victoria Climbié Inquiry. It provides a condensed version of *Working Together* in the form of step-by-step action points and flow charts designed to help front line workers respond appropriately when they suspect abuse and neglect.

Designated and named professionals

The responsibility for child protection services across all health service providers lies with the Primary Care Trusts. They appoint a designated nurse and doctor (usually a senior nurse and a consultant paediatrician) to take the strategic lead in all aspects of the health service contribution to safeguarding children. Designated professionals are responsible for ensuring that policies and procedures are in place and that there are adequate arrangements for consultation, supervision and training. They represent the health service on the local Area Child Protection Committees (ACPCs).

In addition, all NHS trusts must appoint a named doctor and a named nurse/midwife to take the professional lead on child protection matters within their respective trusts and service areas. They are the principal points of contact within health for child protection advice and paediatric opinion and can be consulted about the management of individual cases. In some areas one person will take on the responsibilities of both named and designated professionals in child protection.

What health service workers can do

Anyone may come into contact with or hear about a child who is being harmed and/or an adult who is harming a child. This can happen anywhere and at anytime. Whatever the circumstances, remember child protection is everyone's responsibility. Inquiries into fatal child abuse show that the warning signs are frequently there and known to people both in the wider community as well as the professional network. These reports demonstrate time and time again how important it is that people know what to do if they are concerned about the safety and welfare of a child and how disastrous the outcome can be if they do not.

Working Together to Safeguard Children sets out the parameters of good practice:
- **Be alert to potential indicators of abuse or neglect**
- **Be alert to the risks that individual abusers, or potential abusers, may pose to children**
- **Share and help analyse information so that an informed assessment can be made of the child's needs and circumstances**
- **Contribute to whatever actions are needed to safeguard the child and promote their welfare**
- **Regularly review the outcomes for the child against specific shared objectives**
- **Work co-operatively with parents unless this is inconsistent with the need to ensure the child's safety**

In any encounter with children or families where there is potential, suspected or actual child abuse and/or neglect, assess the child's current situation and needs. Decide whether either of the following is needed:
- **Immediate protection**
- **Urgent medical attention**

If the answer is yes:

- Immediately contact social services or the police and the relevant medical service
- Discuss the concern with the parent/carer and child unless it is considered inappropriate or unsafe to do so – in some circumstances it may place the child at greater risk
- Document in full all details of the incident and the action taken
- Share information with other professionals who know the child/family

If the answer is no:

- Discuss any concerns with the parent/carer unless it is inappropriate or unsafe to do so - in cases of child sexual abuse this may hinder the inquiry and endanger the child
- Listen to the child and document his or her views and feelings
- Check the child/family record for any earlier or on-going concerns.
- Seek advice if necessary from one of the named or designated professionals or other experienced colleague
- Consult colleagues who may know the child/family such as the social worker, general practitioner (GP), health visitor or teacher
- Record full details of the incident/circumstances and all action taken
- Decide whether or not to refer the child to social services.

If a decision is made to refer the child or family to social services, do this in accordance with the local area child protection committee (ACPC) procedures. Discuss concerns with the duty social worker and confirm the referral in writing. Record whether the parent is informed and, if not, why. Always follow up the outcome of any referral to establish that the concern has been understood and is being responded to appropriately. If there is a problem with the response of either the social services, the police or the NSPCC, talk this over with one of the named or designated professionals.

Social services is the lead agency for child protection. It has statutory responsibility for making enquiries into all child protection referrals and for coordinating the inter-agency response. There is a duty to co-operate with any such enquiry and to provide any information relevant to it. As child protection enquiries may reveal other unmet needs, consider any measures taken to safeguard children as part of a wider-ranging assessment of their needs and family circumstances. This is the way to secure the best possible outcome for the child.

Work with children and families cuts across the range of disciplines within the health service, in both primary and secondary care. Remember, therefore, that everyone is part of a multi-disciplinary as well as a multi-agency team. Effective information sharing helps to ensure that all work with vulnerable children is properly coordinated. Research and experience have shown repeatedly that it is only when information from a number of sources has been shared that it becomes clear that a child is at risk of, or is being, harmed.

The paediatric assessment

A child may be referred for a paediatric assessment by a member of the primary health care team, another health professional and/or a professional from another agency, for example social services or education.

Paediatricians can offer an opinion on the medical aspects of abuse and/or neglect. Their expertise enables them to identify the signs of maltreatment in a child. The paediatric assessment is part of the jigsaw that makes up the whole picture; it adds to the information that is being accumulated from the child, family and professional network. Always ensure that the child is referred to a suitably qualified and experienced doctor in order to secure the best assessment available. Consider, too, getting a paediatric opinion on all the children in the family as well as any other children who may be affected.

Forensic medical evidence may be required from children suspected of being sexually abused. In these cases a paediatrician trained in the forensic examination of children, alone or with a forensic medical examiner present (FME), should conduct the assessment.

The function of the paediatric assessment is to:
■ **Confirm the suspicion of non-accidental injury, neglect or sexual abuse and assist in protecting the child by contributing to child**

protection enquiries, and if necessary providing evidence for care or criminal proceedings

■ Verify a diagnosis of accidental injury

■ Identify any medical problem that may cause the symptoms or signs or co-exist with abuse and neglect

■ Provide the child with an opportunity to be seen in their own right and, if they are old enough, to ask questions of the doctor

■ Inform and reassure the child and family about the long-term consequences of any injury – particularly in cases of child sexual abuse

■ Provide follow-up medical support to deal with new signs and symptoms that may have arisen out of continued abuse, symptoms related to any previous injury or in the case of sexual abuse, infections.

■ Monitor any improvement or deterioration in the child's health

■ Ensure the child has access to health care that is not necessarily abuse related, e.g. child and family consultation service

■ Consider the safety and welfare of siblings and their need for assessment

$$\boxed{2}$$

Partnership, collaboration and co-operation

Partnership with parents and children

THE CHILDREN ACT 1989 and *Working Together to Safeguard Children* both stress the value of working openly and collaboratively with families. Indeed, the participation and involvement of parents and children is one of the underlying principles of the Act. Protection from and future prevention of child abuse is achievable by enabling the parents/carers to take good enough care of their own children. Parents have a central role in their children's protection and welfare and should therefore be party, wherever possible, to all decisions and actions relating to them. The outcome for the child is improved if the parent is enabled to participate in all stages of the child protection process.

Ensure that the wishes and feelings of the child, as far as age and understanding permit are heard and accounted for in plans for their future care. Children have a right to know and a need to understand the process through which concerns are raised about their safety. They should be informed and consulted about those actions and decisions that affect them; their views and feelings acknowledged and taken into account. Be sensitive to and considerate of the impact of the family background, culture, religion, ethnicity and class when reviewing a child's physical, emotional and educational needs.

The aim of partnership is to work together to safeguard and promote the welfare of a child. Where this is not possible, or at times when such attempts have failed, social services and/or the police can use their statutory powers to protect the child's interests and welfare. This may be necessary where it is apparent that immediate protection or a more secure framework for long-term safety, health, development and well being is desirable.

There will be instances in which it is not possible to share professional concerns for a child with the parent/carer. This may be either because the parent is not available or because there is a feeling that the child's safety or that of the health professional might be further compromised by doing so. Whatever the reason, respond promptly to the child's need for protection, even if a referral has to be made without the knowledge or consent of the parent/carer. Any delay may jeopardize the child's safety and put them at greater risk.

To challenge a parent about the care of their child is never easy. Making concerns known may introduce a fear of compromising the relationship with the parent/carer. None the less never collude with parents over aspects of care that might threaten the child's safety and welfare. The working partnership is never about collusion and should always operate in the interests of the child.

Inter-agency collaboration and co-operation

It is vital that professionals in all disciplines and within all agencies work together to ensure that the child is protected, and that services for children and their families are properly coordinated. It is only possible to safeguard children effectively if all health workers are committed to working collaboratively with others as part of a multi-agency as well as a multi-disciplinary team.

Everyone must be clear about their own role and understand the part played by colleagues in other disciplines and agencies. Appreciate how information sharing on a 'needs to know' basis is essential for successful inter-agency work. Many communication problems between individuals and agencies arise from a lack of understanding and clarity about roles and responsibilities.

In order to secure the best possible outcomes for children not only must everyone's role be respected and understood but there should also be a willingness to work collaboratively, sharing relevant information to a joint end: the provision of a comprehensive and coordinated service for vulnerable children.

Anti-discriminatory practice

Child-rearing practices are highly diverse, influenced as they are by differences in culture, religion, class, ideology and sexuality. The Children Act 1989 enshrines in its legislation the consideration of a child's needs within this context. The business of anti-discriminatory practice is to ensure that all difference is valued and understood. Judgements about the care and protection of a child have to be based on an objective assessment of facts, and not on assumptions or stereotyped views of divergent cultural values and styles of parenting.

Child abuse and neglect exist within all communities and all cultures. Never condone abuse and neglect or collude with it to avoid being labelled racist. An anti-racist stance that is culturally sensitive must not mean that children from minority ethnic communities receive a lower level of care and protection. If parental behaviour is perceived as harmful, challenge it, but do so sensitively and not in a way that compounds disadvantage. Many families have experienced discriminatory and/or insensitive services at one time or another. Ensure that help is provided in a manner that does not discriminate further but positively promotes the safety and well being of all children.

Area child protection committees (ACPCs)

Local Area Child Protection Committees were established following the Children Act 1989, their aim the coordination and promotion of effective inter-agency work. Every local authority is required to have an Area Child Protection Committee (ACPC), made up of all agencies with responsibility for services to children. Social Services (the lead agency) Health, Education, Police, Probation and the Voluntary Sector are all represented on the ACPC. Within each main agency a number of different services is represented; everyone involved has joint responsibility for contributing to the work of the ACPC.

The purpose of the ACPC is to ensure that services for children in need of protection are properly coordinated; that the inter-agency arrangements for safeguarding and promoting their welfare work effectively and secure the best outcome for them. ACPCs should not just contribute to but also work within the framework established by the local Children's Services Plans.

The ACPC is essentially a management committee. It delegates much of its work to a series of sub-committees, whose membership reflects the diversity of services and agencies involved in child protection. The number and format of the sub-committees may vary among local authorities. However, they will usually include a policy subcommittee, responsible for the development and review of child protection policy and practice, and a training subcommittee, responsible for the provision of multi-agency training. Some ACPCs also contribute to the prevention of maltreatment and the development of support for children in need.

The ACPC is also responsible for reviewing cases of abuse in which a child has died (fatal child abuse) or suffered serious injury. These cases should meet the criteria for case reviews set out in Chapter 8 of *Working Together to Safeguard Children*. The ACPC ensures that lessons are learnt from such tragedies, with changes incorporated into the practice of agencies in the future.

Each ACPC has an up-to-date procedure manual, which details the local procedures that individuals and agencies must follow when abuse is identified. It describes not only how referral works locally but also how each stage of the child protection process is managed. The local procedures should reflect and be consistent with the guidance in *Working Together to Safeguard Children*. They should include inter-agency protocols to deal with specific issues, for example children abused through prostitution.

To ensure the smooth running of inter-agency work, access the ACPC procedure manual and become familiar with its content. Everyone is expected to follow ACPC procedures and work within the framework established by *Working Together to Safeguard Children*. This way, child protection practice works to the best advantage of the child.

Risk assessment

A BUSE OCCURS WHENEVER there is a substantial failure of one person to act towards another with the care appropriate to their relationship. Adults have a duty of care in many aspects of life, both at work and at home, and society expects them to exercise that obligation responsibly and safely. The closer and more dependent the relationship (and they don't get much closer than that of the parent–child), the greater the responsibility to provide care and the greater the risk to the child if care is not provided.

Parental care

Judgements about what does and does not constitute reasonable care are crucial; decisions about the actual or likely risk to a child depend on them. While the Children Act 1989 does not define what it means by reasonable parental care, there is broad agreement that it should include:
- **Provision of adequate nurture**
- **Maintenance of physical health**
- **Protection from violence and abuse**
- **Adequate communication and emotional responsiveness**
- **Adequate expectations to achieve socialisation**

While some forms of abuse are clearly damaging, for example withholding food from a child, other abuse may be less obvious and more difficult to define. Judgements about whether a child is at risk depend on views of what does and does not constitute acceptable care and opinions about this vary over time and across cultures. While it is important to be sensitive to the wide diversity of parenting styles that exist, remember to keep the focus on the child when deciding whether parental behaviour is harmful. Parental care can be placed on a continuum from optimal at one end to unacceptable at the other. Thinking about it in this way may help in assessing the risk to a child and deciding if, when and how to intervene.

A parent may demonstrate:
- Consistent love, warmth and attention. There is appropriate concern, a desire to protect the child from harm, an understanding of the child's needs and feelings and pride in their achievements.
- Responsiveness to the child's needs with intermittent difficulties in relationships and expectations. This may lead to some problems in the child's health, development and/or behaviour.
- Critical or neglectful behaviour showing a poor understanding of and response to the child. This may lead to withdrawn, over-dependent or aggressive behaviour in the child.
- Hostility, cruelty and rejection. Failure to meet the child's basic needs, including the need for emotional responsiveness, leading to significant harm in many aspects of their physical and mental health.

Predisposing factors

To prevent the unnecessary suffering of children, attempt to identify the influences and complex processes that can lead to parenting difficulties and abuse. Consider why some parents and some children are more vulnerable than others, in the sense that they are more likely to abuse or become victims.

None of the predisposing factors that follows has a clear causal link with child abuse. However, there are characteristics common to abusing families, abusing parents and abused children. For any preventive strategy to work give special attention to those parents in the greatest need of help and support. The following pointers will help.

FAMILIES may be vulnerable if there is:
- **Drug and alcohol misuse**
- **Current family violence**

- Previous history of family violence or abuse
- Frequent moves, homelessness
- Social isolation, weak supportive networks of family and friends
- Socio-economic problems, such as poverty and unemployment
- Diffuse social problems
- Poor compliance with professionals

PARENTS/CARERS may be vulnerable if they have:
- Mental health problems, personality disorder
- Unrealistic expectations of child, intolerant and/or indifferent
- Negative perceptions e.g. child miserable, difficult to control
- Little or no ante-natal and post-natal care
- Learning difficulties
- Poor physical health or disability
- A history of abuse and neglect
- No support, e.g. lone parent
- A teenage pregnancy

Consider the impact of a combination of different risk factors. If drug use coexists with domestic violence, for example, the risk to the child may increase considerably. This risk is also compounded if a family refuses to respond to agency intervention. Those who deny the problem, reject help and avoid the involvement of professionals are the most difficult to assist and the most resistant to change. Whatever the source or form of the original abuse, the poor outcomes for many children are often the result of continued inadequate parenting.

CHILDREN may be vulnerable if there is a history of:
- Prematurity and low birth weight
- Separation from mother/principal carer
- Disability
- Multiple birth (e.g. twins) and/or less than 18 months between siblings
- Born different to expectations, for example the wrong sex
- Born unwanted and/or unplanned
- Being looked after
- Not attending school

The exception can disprove the rule. There are always families where risk factors are present, but no abuse. The opposite is also true: serious abuse sometimes occurs in the absence of any of the established predictive factors. A full understanding of why abuse happens in some vulnerable families but not in others can best be gained by looking at its context. Consider abuse in the light of family history, individual characteristics of parents and children, social and environmental circumstances, health problems, life events and chance crises. Understanding the factors that create stress within families helps plan prevention, so that help and support can be given before it occurs.

Assessing risk

Although certain factors seem to highlight a predisposition to abuse, reality is never so clear. While the abuse may be triggered by a single event or isolated crisis, it is likely to be associated with other long-term difficulties. Every incidence of child maltreatment is part of a complex history along a road that leads to the current problem; something that may have begun years before the child was first harmed. The baton of abuse is often passed on from generation to generation. Consider, therefore, not only the immediately obvious but also the less evident and see it in a wider context, as part of the bigger picture.

In assessing the degree of risk to a child from abuse or neglect, consider its severity and duration and any consequences (both actual and likely) for the child's health and development. Consider too the parents'/carers' response to professional concerns. Is there is a history of concern? Use professional judgement to decide whether or not the situation has reached the threshold for a referral to social services and a formal child protection enquiry. Make a decision about if, when and how to intervene. With the impact or consequences of abuse not always immediately obvious, this can be a complicated process. Some effects are immediate and evident; others more hidden and enduring. Share concerns with other experienced colleagues to make these difficult judgements and decisions easier.

$$\boxed{4}$$

Recognition of child maltreatment

T HERE ARE A number of ways in which health care workers may
become aware that a child is either being abused or is potentially
at risk.

Observation Through direct observation of symptoms and signs of
abuse and neglect as demonstrated by both child and parent/carer.
Allegation As a consequence of allegations or reports made by a child
or another person.
Disclosure Either directly from a child or by someone who says they are
harming a child.

Assessing harm

The Children Act 1989 introduced the notion of harm to describe the
various forms and consequences of child maltreatment. Harm covers
impaired health and development and is defined as 'the state of a child
which is attributable to ill-treatment or failure to provide adequate care'.
It includes forms of ill treatment, classified, according to the guidance of
Working Together to Safeguard Children, as:
■ Physical abuse
■ Emotional abuse
■ Sexual abuse
■ Neglect

Whatever the source or nature of harm, professional judgements have to be made about whether the harm to a child is significant enough to reach the threshold to justify a formal child protection enquiry. Significant harm describes the degree of harm caused by ill treatment or the absence of a reasonable standard of parental care. A single event may constitute significant harm, for example a violent assault. However, its impact and extent can perhaps be best understood as 'a compilation of events, both acute and long-standing, which interrupt, change or damage the child's physical and psychological development' (*Working Together*, 1999). Being the victim of significant harm is therefore likely to have a considerable effect both on the child's view of themselves and on their future lives.

As well as bringing together a wide range of possible acts of commission and omission, types of abuse overlap. Clearly, a child who is physically harmed will also suffer emotionally; sexual abuse sometimes involves physical coercion as well as emotional damage; children physically abused may also suffer sexual abuse. In a parenting environment high in criticism and low in warmth, the source of significant harm for the child is likely to be from more than one form of abuse. For this reason the term 'child maltreatment' is used more frequently now to describe all forms of child abuse and neglect. This is in line with the growing recognition that there are more similarities than differences in its various characteristics and manifestations.

When making an assessment remember that harm is not simply a product of poor parental care. Children exposed, for example, to extreme poverty, inadequate housing or bullying at school are less likely to fulfil their optimum potential and develop into happy, healthy and competent adults. Those who suffer from chronic illness and/or disability are less likely to achieve or maintain a reasonable standard of health and development without the provision of a wide range of support services. They may not be in need of protection but they are 'children in need' as described in the Children Act 1989.

Always consider the wider needs of children and families whether or not concerns about maltreatment have been substantiated. Consider too any special needs, such as a communication difficulty, that may affect the child's development and care within the family. Use the assessment framework (see Appendix 1) to consider the child's safety and welfare within the context of their family and wider community. The framework provides all professionals with a systematic way of collecting and analysing information that will help identify whether a child's health and development is being, or may be, affected by their present circumstances. Use it to gain an understanding of:

- a child's developmental needs
- the capacity of parents and carers to respond appropriately to those needs
- the impact of wider family and environmental factors on both the child and parent.

5

Physical abuse

PHYSICAL ABUSE IS potentially serious. It starts, at one end of the continuum, with minor injuries or bruising, and ends at the other with injuries that can prove fatal. Physical abuse is thought to be responsible for the death of approximately 200 children a year in the UK. Its dangers relate closely to age: the younger the child the more at risk they are from physical harm. A baby who has been shaken, for example, can suffer severe and irreversible damage (Shaken Baby Syndrome); even a small bruise in an infant may be a predictor of more severe or possibly fatal abuse.

Most societies condone the use of physical chastisement to discipline children and it remains widespread across all social classes and cultures, involving children of all ages. While there is a difference between physical chastisement and physical abuse it is clear that the two are closely linked. Punishment can be abusive. Many parents who physically abuse their children often begin by disciplining them. Injury results when what they perceive as 'normal' parenting gets out of hand.

An injury that results from failure to protect or provide proper adult supervision can be physically just as damaging. Deliberately placing a child in danger can reflect ambivalent feelings, or a conscious or, indeed, unconscious urge to hurt: leaving an unsupervised toddler in a bath full of water is but one example of how parental neglect can put the child at risk of physical injury.

Be aware of the link between child abuse and domestic violence. The physical abuse of women and children frequently coexist and can begin in pregnancy; if one is present, the other should be suspected.

DEFINITION

Physical abuse is violence directed towards children. *Working Together to Safeguard Children* describes it as possibly involving:

Hitting, shaking, throwing, poisoning, burning or scalding, drowning, suffocating, or otherwise causing physical harm to a child. Physical harm may also be caused when a parent or carer feigns the symptoms of, or deliberately causes ill health to a child whom they are looking after. This situation is commonly described using terms such as factitious illness by proxy or Munchausen syndrome by proxy (now known as Fabricated or Induced Illness, FII).

SIGNS AND SYMPTOMS

Most serious physical abuse occurs in early childhood because of the inability of the immature child to protect themselves. However trivial the injury, remain alert to any signs of physical violence to children: the severity of an injury is only a partial guide to any danger to the child's life and health; even apparently minor problems sometimes signal something more acute. Vigilance is vital and often other abuse co-exists.

IN THE CHILD

■ Injuries of different ages at different stages of healing indicating a series of injuries
■ Certain patterns of injury, such as bruising to a young baby, cigarette burns and fractures in infants and toddlers
■ Frequent minor injuries, scratches and abrasions for which there is no adequate explanation
■ Presence of other signs of abuse, such as neglect, failure to thrive and sexual abuse
■ Sites of bruising that are particularly unlikely to be accidental, e.g. inner thigh, head and trunk
■ Child discloses abuse
■ Injuries not consistent with the explanation given by the child
■ Not accompanied by parent/carer
■ Appears fearful/wary of adults

IN THE PARENT/CARER
- Injuries that are inconsistent with the explanation given by the parent, that is, too many, too severe, the wrong kind, wrong distribution or wrong developmental age
- Unusual behaviour in the parent/carer, such as delay in seeking medical advice, unusual lack of concern, refusal/reluctance to allow treatment, hostile response or over-friendliness towards professionals
- Parent/carer who attributes the cause of the injury to a third party
- Unexplained injury noticed by others, such as at day nursery or school
- History of abuse and/or neglect, domestic violence

CHARACTERISTIC INJURIES

Bruises occur in many physically abused children and can arise from:
- Slapping, pinching or poking
- Use of straps, sticks, buckles or other implements
- Throwing, swinging or pushing on to a hard object
- Adult human bites
- Gripping with or without violent shaking

Multiple bruises may indicate abuse. Bruises at different stages suggest harm may have been inflicted on different occasions, with evidence of different stages of resolution.

The site of the bruising can be meaningful; injuries to the head, eyes, ears and mouth in particular should be viewed with suspicion. Bruising around the neck can suggest suffocation. Bruises below the elbow and knee generally carry less significance than those found on the thighs and upper arms. Those to the trunk (chest and abdomen) tend to indicate abuse, with any to the lower abdomen suggestive of sexual abuse. Bruises on the buttocks, lower back and outer thighs are often punishment related. Injuries to the inner thigh and genital area may suggest either sexual abuse or punishment for perceived toileting misdemeanours, such as bed wetting or lapses in toilet training.

Fractures represent serious injury. They can result from falls and/or extreme violence and may be seen with other injuries, particularly soft-tissue damage. The fracture that follows abuse may be single or multiple, recent or old, or a combination of any of these and found in one or more sites on the body. When an injury is the consequence of abuse the history given by the parent/carer may be vague, inconsistent or non-existent. Medical attention is very often sought after a period of delay when the fracture has caused symptoms such as swelling or loss of function.

Burns and scalds to children are common. While many result from accidents caused by varying degrees of parental neglect, some involve deliberate abuse. Presentation can be as any one of the following:
- Acute injury
- Healed burn or scar
- Neglected or old injury

Delay or avoidance of treatment may occur. Denial of the injury is also an important diagnostic clue. Some parents do not accept responsibility as they may feel that the child deserved what happened and even blame them for it. Always view parental hostility towards the child as suspicious.

While self-inflicted burns or scalds are rare, they are likely to be a sign of extreme disturbance in an abused child.

POISONING

Accidental poisoning of children is a major child health issue in the UK, especially with toddlers aged between two and four years old. However, view repeated ingestion of medicine, tablets or liquids as neglectful and consider the possibility of deliberate poisoning. Whether due to accident, neglect or wilful intent on the part of the parent/carer there is a considerable overlap in the clinical presentation. However, the more bizarre the clinical picture the greater the likelihood of intentional poisoning.

SUFFOCATION

In an infant, suffocation is difficult to detect as a form of abuse because in spite of the violence of the act there is often no sign of injury, even at autopsy. Most sudden and unexpected deaths in infancy are categorised as 'Sudden Infant Death Syndrome' (SIDS), a diagnosis that may conceal abuse, especially if a child in the family has died before in unusual or suspicious circumstances or from SIDS. Include possible suffocation or the Fabrication or Induction of Illness in a child by a carer, in the differential diagnosis of recurrent apnoeic spells in a new baby.

FABRICATED OR INDUCED ILLNESS BY CARERS (FII)

A condition in which a parent/carer, usually the mother, exaggerates or fabricates symptoms and/or causes illness in a child. They may actively intervene in their child's medical treatment, secretly administer drugs or other poisonous substances or smother the child, which can cause apnoea, fits and even death. The mother has a need for recognition of ill health in her child. She repeatedly brings the child, for medical assessments and treatment, often resulting in multiple medical procedures and opinions but no diagnosis. FII can coexist with disability, medical conditions and other types of abuse and neglect. Emotional abuse is also a feature and any distress due to the fabrication or induction of an illness will be further compounded for the child by the invasive medical investigations and associated hospital admissions.

Medical guidance

The following guidelines elaborate on the previous section and should be read with the paediatric assessment (Appendix 2). They are aimed at doctors involved specifically in the diagnosis and management of physical abuse. However, they may be informative to any professional.

ABDOMINAL INJURY

Suspect abdominal injury in a child presenting in poor condition or shock. There may be other injuries, e.g. head and limbs, but no signs of bruising or other external injury. Denial of trauma and delay in presentation adds to the diagnosistic difficultly. Types of injuries include perforation of the gut, haemorrhage, laceration, contusion and haematoma of the organs.

BRAIN, EYE OR OTHER INTERNAL INJURY

Injury to the head and brain is the most common cause of death in childhood. Violently shaking a small child can cause all types of intracranial haemorrhages as well as retinal haemorrhages. Signs include irritability, vomiting, drowsiness, fits and, in extreme cases, unconsciousness. Throwing can cause an impact injury; signs may include fractures of the skull and other bones, and sometimes bruising. Other internal injuries can be present without visible external signs of bruising and may be indicated by vomiting, extreme pallor, fever and severe pain. A combination of these signs can be indicative of Shaken Baby Syndrome.

BRUISING

Bruising may be variable in size and colour, old or new, or unexplained, and be found anywhere on the body. If there are bruises on the face, mouth, ear or side of the head in a baby or young child, check for accompanying internal head injury, which could be life threatening. Remember that bruising at a site not usually or easily injured is always suspicious, such as to the head and neck, which may be caused by strangulation. Suspect sexual abuse when bruising is seen on the trunk, thighs or abdomen. Injury to the genital area may be due to sexual abuse or perceived toilet misdemeanours. Any bruising on the buttocks and/or lower back may be punishment associated.

SUSPICIOUS SIGNS

- Any bruises to an infant or child, especially on non-bony prominences, on the trunk, abdomen, cheek, the head or to the ears. Purple ear or petechial bruising usually occurs on the upper half of the ear, from blows or pinching
- Any lacerations or bruising in and around the mouth, especially if the frenulum is torn (the frenulum is the bridge of tissue that joins the middle of the inside top lip to the gum)
- Finger-tip bruising (small, round or oval marks indicating gripping), slap or punch marks (note imprint of hand, ring, knuckle, etc.)
- Bruising from adult human bite marks (in the shape of two crescents). If more than 3cm across, this must have been caused by an adult or older child with permanent teeth (a forensic dental opinion may be necessary)
- Linear bruises or outlines of weapons such as sticks, belts or other instruments (the weapon's shape may be clearly etched on the skin)
- Evidence of multiple bruising, either old or new and of various colours

Do not confuse Mongolian blue spots with bruising. These are birthmarks common to children of African, Caribbean, Asian or Chinese ethnicity, and can occur in 'white' children.   They are dark blue and often look similar to a fading bruise; they last for several months and even years after birth. They feature mainly on the back or the buttocks but can be seen anywhere on the body.

BURNS AND SCALDS

Make a decision about whether or not a burn is accidental in the light of a child's age and development and in the context of the explanation given by the child and/or their carers. Symptoms may be either acute, or from a neglected or old injury, or even a healed burn or scar. No site is exempt but they commonly include the backs of hands, buttocks, genitalia and feet. Burns maybe associated with all other forms of abuse including sexual abuse. Skin allergies, infection, birthmarks and old scars all resemble burns, but the deliberate burn is more likely to be regular in shape with a clear outline.

SUSPICIOUS SIGNS

- Burns to the lips and surrounding skin, sometimes including the inside of mouth
- Burns to the backs of the hands, feet and genitalia (accidental burns are more likely on the palms of the hands and soles of the feet)
- Cigarette burns seen as small circular areas of skin loss that vary in size from 6mm to 2cm depending on pressure and duration. Accidental brushing against a cigarette end rarely makes such marks and usually results in a 'tail'. Not to be confused with impetigo and healed chicken pox scars
- Contact burns are caused by holding a hot object such as electric fire, poker or iron against a child's skin. The margins are delineated, reflecting the pattern of the object, and the depth is usually uniform
- Radiant burns are usually extensive in a limited area and can be caused by standing too close to a fire
- Friction burns can be caused by dragging a child across a carpet or from restraining them with a tie, e.g. a rope
- Immersion burns from dipping a child into hot water tend to be uniform over all exposed areas with clear demarcation lines. View absence of splash marks as suspicious
- Splash burns from hot water thrown at or poured over a child

DEATH OF A SIBLING

If a child is admitted with an unclear diagnosis, and a child or a sibling is known to have died previously also with an equally unsatisfactory explanation or diagnosis, undertake a careful, thorough medical investigation. If still suspicious, refer to social services as filicide is a possible cause.

DELIBERATE POISONING

Depending on the history of the type of poison and the quantity ingested, there may be drowsiness and unsteadiness, and other symptoms such as fits, hyperventilation and coma. Be particularly concerned by any bizarre or unexplained symptoms. Accidental poisoning is more common and occurs most frequently in toddlers aged 2 to 4 years old, who explore and may try out any medicine, tablets or other liquids that they find. None the less accidental ingestion, especially if repeated, may be a sign of neglect or wilful intent to harm.

DROWNING

Drowning can result from extreme negligence and is therefore not always accidental, e.g. leaving a child unattended in a bath. Children who are deliberately drowned may have other signs of abuse.

FABRICATED OR INDUCED ILLNESS BY CARERS (FII)

This condition includes a wide spectrum of problems that are fabricated and/or induced in a child by a parent/carer. The child repeatedly presents for medical assessments and treatment, often resulting in multiple medical procedures and opinions but no diagnosis. Although the perpetrator denies any knowledge of the cause of the child's condition, the signs and symptoms cease when the child is separated from the perpetrator.

WARNING SIGNS

- Unexplained signs and reported symptoms, despite extensive medical investigation
- Treatment does not produce the expected effect
- Symptoms and signs that only occur in the presence of the parent
- Presence of unexplained illnesses, death or multiple surgery in other family members
- Withdrawal of special treatment (e.g. naso-gastric feeds, intra-venous lines), and 'getting better' not viewed with enthusiasm by the parents/carers
- Repeat presentations to a variety of doctors with a variety of problems
- Specific problems such as apnoea, fits
- Child's daily activities curtailed more than expected

Be wary of situations that put the child at risk of significant harm:
- Parent/carer causes illness in the child by administration of noxious substances, for example laxatives (low toxicity) and salt, drugs (high toxicity)
- High level of demand for multiple (unnecessary and at the time possibly dangerous) investigations because of the parent's belief that the child is ill
- Active withholding of food or the giving of insufficient food so that the child fails to thrive
- Verbal fabrication and production of signs such as fever
- Apparent Life Threatening Events (ALTE), including smothering

Be aware how this can impair the child's physical and emotional development by:
- Exposing them to unnecessary, harmful and painful investigations or treatment
- Social isolation/over-protection because of supposed symptoms
- Missing school
- Confusion about their own health and illness

Apart from certain clear exceptions, multi-agency assessment and psychiatric evaluation are the next likely course of action.

FRACTURES

Any fracture in the first year of life, with no clear accidental history, is of immediate concern; immobile babies rarely break their bones accidentally.   Such fractures may present with pain, swelling and/or unwillingness to use the affected part, though confirmation by X-ray is essential.   Refer for a CT or ultrasound scan to exclude intracranial injury in a child under one year and consider these investigations in a child over one year of age. Twisting and pulling, a direct blow, shaking or squeezing a limb resulting in a fracture may or may not be associated with bruising and other external signs. Fractures can be a presenting feature in genetic, metabolic and other bone disease, such as osteogenesis imperfecta and osteomyelitis.

SUSPICIOUS SIGNS

- Rib fractures – single or mutliple are common in abused infants, and strongly suggest squeezing, shaking, kicking or blows
- Metaphyseal-epiphyseal fractures
- Formation of new periosteal new bone
- Skull fracture with intracranial injury
- Shaft fractures may result from direct blows, bending and violent pulling to long bones
- Single fractures, often spiral, with and without multiple bruising
- Multiple fractures at different stages of healing in the presence of normal bones
- Evidence of old fractures
- Unusual fractures, e.g. scapula

TYPES

- GREENSTICK FRACTURES, in which the bone cracks half-way across and splits some way up its length resulting in an incomplete break; they are often accidental
- SPIRAL FRACTURES are due to a twisting force, such as being swung by the arms or legs; highly suggestive of abuse in immobile children
- METAPHYSEAL FRACTURES, in which fragments of the bone become separated from the distal ends of long bones, either as a chip or a whole plate, and show up on X-ray in the shape of a 'bucket-handle'. The force disrupts the fine layer of new bone close to its junction with the cartilage. Such injuries are usually from gripping and twisting movements and shaking. Usual sites affected: elbows, knees, wrists and ankles. There may be soft tissue swelling initially and little pain, tenderness or swelling after the injury
- LONG BONE FRACTURES may result from violent pulling, gripping or twisting injuries and do not always have external signs
- PERIOSTEAL NEW BONE FORMATION. The periosteum is a thin layer of bone that protects the long bones in the arms and legs. Damage caused by gripping or twisting injuries raises it from the shaft of the bone and new bone appears 7–10 days later

SUDDEN UNEXPECTED DEATH IN INFANCY

Any sudden unexpected and unexplained death requires thorough investigation including a post-mortem and the police, social services and the coroners are always notified. Ensure a paediatric pathologist undertakes the post-mortem when the death appears suspicious or there is a history of sudden infant death syndrome (SIDS) in the family. Differential diagnosis includes SIDS, infection, cardiac or pulmonary disorder, suffocation, poisoning, shaken baby syndrome and FII.

SUFFOCATION

Consider deliberate suffocation in any acute life-threatening episode, especially if multiple and/or familial. There may not be external signs of injury but where they occur include hand marks, multiple petechiae, bruising (especially on the face) and bleeding from the mouth or nose.

6

Sexual abuse

CHILD SEXUAL ABUSE is devastating for children, for boys as much as for girls. It is a major cause of morbidity in children and adults. The outlook for victims of child sexual abuse is bleak if the abuse is not identified at an early stage as they may be then at risk of abuse for years and could be vulnerable to other perpetrators. Recognition of child sexual abuse and protection of its victims depends on the willingness of adults to acknowledge that the abuse might be happening, to listen to and believe the child and take appropriate action in response to what they are being told.

DEFINITION

Child sexual abuse is the sexual molestation of children by adults or older children (sexual, here meaning any activity that leads to sexual arousal in the perpetrator). The abuse may range from voyeurism and exhibitionism to oral, vaginal or anal penetration. It may be perpetrated by single or multiple perpetrators, on one or more occasions, and associated with other types of abuse. *Working Together to Safeguard Children* describes it as:

> Forcing or enticing a child or young person to take part in sexual activities, whether or not the child is aware of what is happening. The activities may involve physical contact, including penetrative (e.g. rape or buggery) or non-penetrative acts. They may include non-contact activities, such as involving children in looking at pornographic material or watching sexual activities, or encouraging children to behave in sexually inappropriate ways.

ESSENTIAL CHARACTERISTICS

These can be summarised as follows:

- Responsibility rests entirely with the perpetrator
- Sexual gratification of the perpetrator is the usual aim of the abuse
- Power/age gap means the child cannot refuse
- It is usually secretive and collusive
- Children in general do not like it and want it to stop, although their need for physical affection and attention can sometimes lead to their apparent complicity or willingness to initiate and maintain the abuse

The element of force or coercion is an important one. While some abuse is clearly the result of violent acts resulting in physical injury, the majority of sexually abused children are victims of a more cautious if equally determined approach that involves the use of threats, bribes and emotional manipulation. In determining whether the activity is abusive, remember that the issue of coercion relates closely to age difference. Distinguish between normal sexual development in children, for example the mutually exploratory sexual play of pre-school children, and sexual activity that involves coercion. Sexual abuse is an abuse of power and as such can be perpetrated by adults, children and young people, of both genders.

PATTERNS OF ABUSE

In the majority of cases the perpetrator is known to the child and is probably a family member. He is more likely to be male than female, although sexual abuse by women is now increasingly recognised. Child sexual abuse crosses social and cultural groups, affecting children of all ages, including babies. Boys are less likely to report abuse than girls.

When abuse occurs within the nuclear and extended family it is described as 'intra-familial'. When it involves other adults known to the child from a variety of sources, it is termed 'extra-familial'. When it happens within institutions: 'institutional'. When it is the result of a random attack in a public place or the abduction of a child: 'stranger abuse'. In addition some children are abused through prostitution. Some groups of people form paedophile rings and the use of the internet to develop such networks is well recognised.

Sexual abuse occurs when the perpetrator has access to an available and vulnerable child. As it is a secretive activity the family can offer a safe outlet. Within it, the child can be controlled and manipulated into silence and any risk of discovery minimised. Intra-familial abuse may involve a pattern of relationships in which there is collusion with other members of the family, where the normal boundaries within and between generations do not exist.

Intra-familial and extra-familial abuse may co-exist, so if one is present, the other should be considered. Perpetrators deliberately target families where they think the abuse is likely to remain undetected. In extra-familial abuse the adult, usually known to the child, forms a relationship with them to lure them into situations in which abuse can take place, sometimes in return for attention or something the child is not getting at home.

PHYSICAL INDICATORS

Physical indicators of child sexual abuse are important as they may be the only signs of abuse in infants and young children or in older children not able to communicate. For the child who discloses abuse such signs can help corroborate their story. None the less, a normal physical examination must not exclude the possibility of child sexual abuse. Healing takes place rapidly, and scarring is uncommon so be aware that many children who have been sexually abused show no physical signs.

Injury and/or infection can be a consequence of physical interference with the child's genitalia, anus or mouth. Principal symptoms of injury are pain, soreness, swelling and bleeding. Symptoms of infection include vaginal discharge and soreness. Irritation of the urethra causes dysuria and frequency of micturition. Sexual and physical abuse are intimately linked; some sexually abused children are also abused physically. With the exception of pregnancy, some sexually transmitted diseases and/or the presence of sperm in the vagina or rectum, a single physical sign may support the diagnosis of child sexual abuse but is rarely diagnostic.

BEHAVIOURAL INDICATORS

Children who are abused sexually are often groomed and trained, so the process occurs over several months or years. Consequently, a child sometimes displays behaviour that may be perceived as contributing to or even precipitating the abuse; they seem to encourage or provoke a sexual response in the perpetrator. View these behavioural signs as the consequence of the abuse rather than its cause.

Over time children can develop a pattern of adjustment to the abuse, displaying characteristics such as:

Secrecy Children are told not to tell. Threats of withdrawal of love and affection, fear of punishment and/or fear of not being believed are often all that is needed to secure a child's cooperation

Helplessness Children in most cases are not able to stop the abuse. They give up resisting to protect themselves

Self-blame Children hold themselves responsible for the abuse. Self-blame and guilt are almost universal feelings

Delayed disclosure Many children never tell; for those that do it is often delayed and understated; it may take place when the abuse has stopped

Retraction This is a frequent response by the child to the disruption of the family and the involvement of professionals

Be aware that because children develop complex coping mechanisms to accommodate the abuse they may appear happy and well. Some seriously sexually abused children show no signs or symptoms at all. Others, however, show disturbed behaviour, such as wetting, soiling, self-injury, running away and/or emotional problems like anxiety, depression and withdrawal. There may be difficulty with learning and under-achievement at school. Relationships with other adults and within their peer group are likely to be affected, which can be expressed in sexualised behaviour towards both adults and other children.

PERPETRATORS

Remember that:

- Most are related or known to the child
- May commit a large number of offences involving a lot of children
- Include both men and women
- May begin their offending behaviour as adolescents
- May have been abused and neglected as children
- High likelihood of re-offending
- Most deny the abuse and refuse to participate in treatment programmes

Once an adult or young person has been convicted of an offence against a child they are classified and become known as 'Schedule 1 Offenders'. This includes all forms of child maltreatment and child murder as well as child sexual abuse. The Sex Offenders Act 1997 requires certain categories of sex offenders, convicted since September 1997, to notify the police of their current whereabouts and any change to it. In this way agencies with child protection responsibilities are able to manage and monitor the risk they present to children.

Medical guidance

The following guidelines elaborate on the previous section and should be read with the paediatric assessment (Appendix 2). They are aimed at doctors involved specifically in the diagnosis and management of child sexual abuse However, they may be informative to any professional.

SYMPTOMS AND SIGNS

Child sexual abuse may present in a variety of ways, some of which clearly indicate the probability of abuse while others lead only to its suspicion. Symptoms and signs are age related, for example the pre-school child may present with sexualised play and the young person with promiscuity. A disclosure by the child is an important pointer to a diagnosis of sexual abuse; false allegation is rare.

Diagnosis should rarely be made on the physical signs alone as more than half of sexually abused children have no abnormalities on examination; remember, absence of physical signs does not imply absence of abuse. The presence of signs varies according to the type of abuse – oral, anal and vaginal – and how long it has been since the most recent episode. As a general rule, be familiar with genital anatomy and always refer to a senior colleague.

There are a few diagnostic signs but consider none the less the different levels of suspicion outlined below. Behavioural changes may co-exist, occur alone or be the presenting problem. Interpret all signs and symptoms in the context of the child's social and other related circumstances.

DIAGNOSTIC SIGNS

- Semen in vagina, anus or on external genitalia
- Pregnancy
- Laceration or scars in the hymen, which may extend to the posterior vaginal wall
- Attenuation of the hymen with loss of hymenal tissue (posteriorly or completely)

- Laceration or healed scar extending beyond the anal mucosa on to the perianal skin
- Sexually transmitted infections outside the relevant incubation period for vertical transmission

SUSPICIOUS SIGNS AND SYMPTOMS

HIGH LEVEL OF SUSPICION
- Allegation/disclosure by child, sibling or another person
- Pregnancy, where the identity of the father is unknown or concealed
- Acute hymenal or anal injury not severe enough to be diagnostic
- Scarring of the posterior forchette
- Bruises, scratches or other acute injuries to the genital or anal areas, or to other 'sexual' areas, such as breasts and lips: these injuries may be minor but are inconsistent with accidental injury
- Repeated and frequent sexualised behaviour

MEDIUM LEVEL OF SUSPICION
- Grossly enlarged hymenal opening greater than 1.5cm
- Anal warts
- Anal laxity without other explanation e.g. chronic constipation
- Reflex anal dilatation that is greater than 1.5cm and reproducible
- Chronic anal changes, multiple anal fissures
- Child hinting that there are secrets about which they cannot talk
- Psychiatric disturbances, mutism, anorexia, deliberate self-harm
- Concern about inappropriate behaviour with other children or adults
- Allegation by another person

LOW LEVEL OF SUSPICION
- Perineal itching, vulvovaginitis, dysuria, vaginal discharge
- Labial fusion
- Recurrent urinary tract infections
- Recurrent abdominal pain, headaches or other psychosomatic features
- Isolated observation of sexualised behaviour

■ 'Eccentric' sexual patterns of family interaction without other observable or reported symptomatology

BEHAVIOURAL PRESENTATIONS

■ Child shows sexualised behaviour through words, play or drawing; or hints at the presence of serious family conflict, family secrets or puzzling and/or uncomfortable things at home but is fearful of intervention (sex-education classes may lead some children suddenly to question what has been happening to them, often over a period of years)

■ Child with an excessive pre-occupation with sexual matters and detailed and precocious knowledge of adult sexual behaviour; one who repeatedly engages in age-inappropriate sexual play/behaviour with peers, adults, toys or themselves

■ Abrupt changes in mood or behaviour including regressive behaviour

■ Enuresis, encopresis – sudden onset or prolonged

■ Changes in eating patterns, such as loss of appetite and faddiness, or excessive pre-occupation with food

■ Loss of self-esteem and desire to make themselves unattractive; depression

■ Lack of trust in familiar adults or marked fear of men

■ Pseudo-mature or overly compliant behaviour, often masking distress and anger

■ Aggressive, attention seeking or poor concentration

■ Social isolation, poor peer relationships

■ Severe sleep disturbance, with fears, phobias, vivid dreams or nightmares, sometimes having overt or veiled sexual content

■ Inappropriate displays of affection between parents and children, including behaviour reminiscent of adult intimacy rather than parent/child intimacy

■ Young people may present with mental health problems, deliberate self-harm. They may make persistent attempts to run away from home; exhibit sexualised behaviour and in some cases may become abused through prostitution. There may be drug and/or alcohol misuse

MANAGEMENT OF SUSPECTED OR ACTUAL CHILD SEXUAL ABUSE

Where there is a high level of suspicion or diagnostic findings, refer the child to a senior experienced paediatrician immediately so they can decide on the best course of action. Forensic specimens can be taken up to seven days after the event; children must not bathe prior to a paediatric forensic medical examination. Sometimes the police will request a paediatric forensic medical examination which needs to be carried out by a forensically trained doctor. The Royal College of Paediatrics and Child Health has produced guidance on the competencies needed to examine such children properly. The examination may be carried out by one or two doctors, depending on their medical expertise (core skills) and the clinical presentation of the child (case-dependent skills).

Where there is a medium or low level of suspicion, GPs, paediatricians and social workers may refer children for a further opinion. Such children do not need to be seen urgently. The paediatrician must include sexual abuse in the differential diagnosis.

Remember all the symptoms and signs of child sexual abuse are part of a wider picture that will inform the multi-agency assessment and planning process needed to protect the child. However, even diagnostic signs may not secure a conviction of a suspected perpetrator in criminal proceedings. While decisions about the safety of children in care proceedings are made on the balance of probabilities, a criminal court has to prove, beyond reasonable doubt, that the accused perpetrator is guilty of the crime.

7

Neglect

Neglect is the most prevalent form of child maltreatment, and now represents up to one half of children and young people on child protection registers in the UK. It is an insidious form of abuse affecting children in a variety of ways, including impaired growth and development, and poor health. Its consequences can be severe and long term, depriving children of the opportunity to realise their potential in all areas of social functioning, relationships and educational achievement. Neglect encompasses emotional deprivation, and there is a risk of physical and sexual abuse as well. It is a contributory factor in many child deaths and in extreme cases it may be the direct cause. *Working Together to Safeguard Children* describes neglect as:

> **The persistent failure to meet a child's basic physical and psychological needs, likely to result in the serious impairment of the child's health and development. It may involve a parent or carer failing to provide adequate food, shelter and clothing, failing to protect a child from physical harm or danger, or the failure to ensure access to appropriate medical care or treatment. It may also include neglect of or unresponsiveness to a child's basic emotional needs.**

KEY FEATURES

With some forms of abuse parents behave in a way that can be perceived as hostile and interfering towards a child. Neglect, however, is defined through acts of parental omission. Sometimes known as 'passive abuse', it is nevertheless a failure to provide or respond to the changing needs of a growing child. The extent of this ranges from the inadequate but well-intentioned efforts of parents with limited intellectual resources, to the detached disinterest of a clinically depressed parent/carer. It can also be expressed in the deliberate deprivation of basic requirements such as food, warmth, protection and affection.

Neglect can involve lack of physical care, limited or non-existent emotional responsiveness, absence of supervision and control, and not seeking or refusing medical care when required. It commonly includes a failure to provide the opportunity for social, emotional and cognitive development. Rarely expressed through a single incident, neglect is usually chronic and the result of a culmination of factors operating over a considerable period of time.

Mental health problems, learning difficulties, substance misuse and poverty feature regularly in the histories of the parents. Their problems are often multiple; further adversity compounds disadvantage, and patterns of disadvantage prevail from generation to generation. These long-term consequences of neglect are known as 'cycles of deprivation'. Many parents who neglect their children lack the skills, resources and motivation to be good enough parents. Neglected children are subsequently at risk of growing up into adults with limited skills and competence, becoming themselves, in turn, inadequate and neglectful parents.

IMPAIRMENT OF HEALTH AND DEVELOPMENT

The impact of neglect varies according to the temperament, characteristics and coping mechanisms of the child. Take this into account when making a connection between neglectful parenting and the child's health and development.

Consider the key symptoms and signs described below as potential indicators of neglect to be added to any other relevant information about the child's and the family's circumstances.

INFANTS: 0–2 YEARS

PHYSICAL   Failure to thrive
Recurrent and persistent minor infections
Frequent accidents
Frequent visits to the GP
Frequent attendance at casualty departments and/or

hospital admissions

Late presentation with physical symptoms

DEVELOPMENT Late attainment of milestones, e.g. pre-linguistic skills

Little or no child health promotion (immunisation and developmental checks)

BEHAVIOUR Attachment disorders: anxious, avoidant, difficult to console

Lack of social responsiveness

Self-stimulatory behaviour – rocking and head banging

The Primary Health Care Team sees infants more regularly than older children, with a greater opportunity therefore to recognise neglect of their physical and emotional care. Neglect may feature in a baby not fed sufficiently or appropriately for their age and failing to thrive. It can feature in an infant who is habitually cold and wet, or has a severe nappy rash, sometimes a sign that nappies are not changed regularly.

PRE-SCHOOL CHILDREN: 2–5 YEARS

PHYSICAL Failure to thrive

Unkempt and dirty, poor hygiene

Frequent accidents

DEVELOPMENT Speech and language delay

Socio-emotional immaturity

BEHAVIOUR Overactive

Aggressive and impulsive

Indiscriminate friendliness

Seek physical contact from strangers

Physical consequences of persistent abuse and neglect through the pre-school period can include poor growth. Language development is especially vulnerable to the effects of a severely depriving environment, frequently compounded by recurrent and inadequately treated middle-ear infections that cause mild to moderate hearing loss.

Peer relations for neglected children can be difficult, as they lack the opportunity to develop the social skills necessary for co-operative play. Some children elicit intimate contact from complete strangers, even in the presence of their primary caregiver, and appear to crave physical contact ('touch hunger').

SCHOOL-AGE CHILDREN: 5–16 YEARS

PHYSICAL	Short stature, variable weight gain
	Poor hygiene, poor general health
	Unkempt appearance
	Underweight or obese
DEVELOPMENT	Mild to moderate learning difficulties
	Low self-esteem
	Poor coping skills
	Socio-emotional immaturity
	Poor concentration
BEHAVIOUR	Disordered or few relationships
	Self-stimulating and/or self-injurious behaviour
	Soiling and wetting
	Conduct disorders, aggressive, destructive and withdrawn
	Poor attendance at school or truanting
	Runaways, delinquent behaviour

In the school-age child the effects and main indicators of long-term abuse and neglect are usually found in poor social and emotional adjustment, behaviour problems and low educational attainment. Schools may not be able to compensate for the long-term lack of cognitive stimulation at home because neglected children have great trouble attending to learning tasks, often exacerbated by poor attendance. Never rule out neglect as a possible cause in children who are disruptive and difficult to manage at school.

As with other forms of abuse recognition and a prompt response to signs of neglect are crucial; the longer neglect continues the more difficult it becomes to influence the outcome for children and their families. However, if neglect is substituted by sensitive care – and this may be in a foster placement or even hospital setting – a rapid and dramatic improvement in growth, developmental progress and behaviour often follows.

8

Emotional abuse

EMOTIONAL ABUSE IS probably the most complex form of abuse to define, recognise and identify. It is under-recognised and frequently viewed as an accompanying or subordinate feature of other forms of abuse. Fewer than 20 per cent of children are placed on child protection registers under the category of emotional abuse, although the emotional consequences of all forms of abuse are likely to be the most damaging.

The impact of continual emotional maltreatment is cumulative, serious and long term. Emotional abuse impairs the child's psychological and emotional development with a potentially life-long influence on any capacity to form successful relationships. In addition child victims often form poor relationships with their own children.

DEFINITION

Emotional development in infancy and later childhood largely depends on 'good enough parenting', which determines the quality of the attachment. Emotional abuse describes a relationship between the parent and child that is characterised by harmful interactions, which impair a child's psychological and emotional health and development; no physical contact is required. The abusing adult is nearly always the primary carer and attachment figure for the child. Different forms of emotional abuse affect children differently according to age and shape the development of psychological function at the time of its occurrence. Often children who are maltreated experience emotional abuse from an early age, frequently as a precursor to other abuse. *Working Together to Safeguard Children* describes emotional abuse as having:

An important impact on a developing child's mental health, behaviour and self esteem. Underlying emotional abuse may be as important, if not more so, than other more visible forms of abuse in terms of its impact on the child.

KEY FEATURES

These are not easy to define precisely. How often and to what degree does a child have to be subjected to verbal abuse, for example, before it becomes damaging?

Sustained and repetitive responses of negative emotion, such as criticism, threats or ridicule convey to children that they are worthless, unloved and unwanted and impair their emotional and psychological development in particular and therefore their welfare in general. Components of emotionally abusive behaviour include the following:

REJECTING refusing to acknowledge the child's worth and the legitimacy of their needs

ISOLATING cutting off the child from normal social experiences and contact with peers or adults

TERRORISING verbally assaulting the child, creating a climate of fear and bullying

IGNORING depriving the child of essential stimulation and emotional responsiveness

CORRUPTING 'mis-socialising' the child, encouraging destructive and antisocial behaviour

Some parents and carers knowingly and deliberately harm their children through emotional abuse in the ways outlined above; for example, some violent men may terrorise a child in order to maintain control and dominance in the family. The majority, however, have no conscious wish to do so and appear in many respects to be quite ordinary parents. None the less, those with mental health problems, those with difficulties that manifest in violent relationships or substance misuse and those with learning difficulties may be unintentionally abusive towards their children. Witnessing violence between parents, for example, is a harmful experience for a child, even though this may not be something deliberate on the part of the parents. They may not even be aware of the impact of their behaviour on the child, which can contribute to professional reluctance to acknowledge the abuse.

Remember, it is the sustained, repetitive and inappropriate parental response that is key to determining the degree of harm/damage to the child. It can be illustrated by the following:

- Emotional unavailability, unresponsiveness and neglect
- Promoting insecure attachment, conditional parenting, inconsistency and unpredictability
- Persistent negative attributions – denigration, belittling, hostility or blaming, child seen as deserving discipline, rejection and punishment
- Inappropriate or inconsistent developmental expectations. Unrealistic expectations of a child, failure to protect and overprotection
- Failure to recognise and acknowledge child's individuality and psychological boundary, an inability to distinguish between child's reality and parents' beliefs and wishes. Using the child to meet parents' own needs
- Failure to promote child's social adaptation or actively mis-socialising

IMPAIRMENT OF HEALTH AND DEVELOPMENT

Children who have been emotionally abused often exhibit high levels of anxiety, and many have an insecure attachment to their primary caregiver. The child's inability to control events and manage their own feelings can result in provocative, aggressive and antisocial behaviour, on the one hand, and despair, depression and withdrawal on the other. Some children are compliant and watchful, eager to please adults in order to avoid further abuse. Others direct their anger and aggression towards themselves.

Emotionally maltreated children generally have very low self-esteem. They experience difficulty in giving and receiving affection and form poor relationships both within their family and at school. They can be punitive to others and lack empathy. Some or all of the following indicators may be expressions of a child's distress at emotional abuse.

CHILD'S AGE

0–1 Sleep/feeding problems, irritability, apathetic, anxious or avoidant attachments to primary caregivers, failure to thrive

1–3 As above PLUS indiscriminate affection, fearful and anxious, aggressive, inability to play, anxious and ambivalent attachments, language delay

3–6 As above PLUS peer-relationship difficulties, attention seeking, clingy, poor performance in school, poor social skills

6–12 As above, although sleep and feeding problems may resolve, inappropriate attachment to carers, rejected by peers, poor school attendance, poor educational attainment, developing delinquent behaviours, running away, truancy, wetting, soiling, stealing, victims as well as perpetrators of bullying

12 As above PLUS depression, escalated aggression, anxiety, self-harm (overdosing), psychosomatic illness, drug and substance misuse, criminal activities, promiscuity

When emotional abuse becomes integral to the relationship between the child and primary caregiver, the child may respond by attempting to minimise the risk of further abuse. An infant's response to an anxious mother may, for example, be to resist eating in order to avoid a traumatic feed, which, in turn, creates greater tension and anxiety in the mother. If this pattern continues the infant may lose weight and become harder to handle, the situation potentially spiralling down into physical abuse, rejection and failure to thrive. A tragic consequence of this downward curve of attachment behaviour is that the attempts of the child to avoid harm may increase the likelihood of further abuse.

Although there is no single event, sign or symptom that characterises emotional abuse, always consider it if the harmful interactions between parent and child are constant and there is serious concern about the child's functioning and emotional state. Unlike sexual abuse which is a secret activity, the quality of the relationship between parent and child is easily observable. Emotional abuse may be hard to identify and manage; but being able to articulate concerns about negative parent/child interactions and show that they are causing significant harm will be crucial in improving the outcome for emotionally abused children.

9

Failure to thrive

FAILURE TO THRIVE describes children who do not adequately gain weight or achieve the expected rate of growth for their age. In addition it includes infants and young children whose length has fallen below the norm. Although mostly used with reference to babies and young children, failure to thrive can persist throughout childhood and into adolescence. If it passes unrecognised and untreated it has potentially adverse consequences for a child's health and development.

Failure to thrive can be organic (a feature of many medical conditions) or non-organic, or a mixture of both. What causes failure to thrive is complex and varied, and there are both genetic and environmental influences. Organic failure to thrive usually has a physiological basis and is associated with inadequate nutrition secondary to gastrointestinal disorders, chronic infection, major structural congenital abnormalities, and metabolic and endocrine defects. Non-organic failure to thrive is also linked to inadequate nutrition, but refers to children whose failure to grow has no underlying medical condition. In some cases it may be accompanied by other concerns about the child's well being and safety. Whatever causal factors are involved, all children who fail to thrive have a less than adequate intake of calories and are therefore not able to grow well.

Organic and non-organic factors commonly co-exist, and the presence of one often leads to the rise of the other. Failure to thrive may be associated with all types of child maltreatment, including emotional abuse and neglect. In some cases poor growth is a marker that signals a child in need of protection as well as a child in need.

Feeding or eating problems are common in children whether they have been maltreated or not. However, some mothers of infants who fail to put on weight experience an acute sense of failure themselves, which may lead to abuse. This may be expressed in behaviour that ranges from indifference and withdrawal (that is, failure to provide adequate/appropriate food, ignoring signals of hunger) to active hostility (such as force-feeding, screaming or smacking) and rejection of the child. The temperament and response of the child can add to the downward spiral of attachment. Children who are often unwell, for example, or difficult to feed, or who cry persistently can provoke a negative response from their parents/carers that makes matters worse. A negative pattern of interaction then develops that, if not interrupted at an early stage, can lead to a further distortion of the parent–child relationship, attachment disorders, developmental impairment and growth failure.

Some infants and children fail to thrive because they are generally under-stimulated and neglected as well as underfed. Parents who lack the capacity or are unwilling to provide adequate physical and emotional care are often unresponsive to their children's needs and show limited concern for their welfare.

PATTERNS OF GROWTH: CRITERIA FOR CONCERN

The distribution of growth parameters – that is weight, height and head circumference – is shown on a growth chart. Growth is usually a smooth, continuous process with small variations around the child's own centile. In general terms the nearer the child is to their own centile, which is usually reached by one year of age, and the more closely they follow it, the more likely they are to be in good health. Most healthy children approximately match height and weight centiles. Consider any deviation in the expected growth trajectory in the light of other information about the child's circumstances. As a guideline, the criteria for poor growth should be applied to all children whose weight deviates downwards across two or more centiles.

Abnormal patterns of growth exist where the:
- **Growth trajectory falls or crosses the centile**
- **Height and weight centiles are markedly discrepant.**

GROWTH TRAJECTORY FALLS OR CROSSES THE CENTILES

The child continues to put on weight although the gain is insufficient for their age and height, as demonstrated by the fall in centile position. If the child loses weight the decline in centile position will be faster. The latter may be due to an acute illness that is followed by recovery and rapid weight gain – 'catch-up growth'.

Many children who fail to thrive cross several centiles over the first few years and then continue to grow along the low height and weight centile that they have reached. In addition some children start life on a low centile, and their poor rate of growth only becomes apparent when their circumstances change and their rate of growth accelerates. It is now thought that some children are able to adapt to a state of poor nutrition that often involves loss of appetite.

If there is a change in the child's circumstances and the level of food intake increases there can be significant change in the growth velocity and an improvement in the centile position – 'catch-up growth'. It is also seen when children are taken into care and the new circumstances of their foster home provoke an acceleration of growth; this is known as a 'retrospective rise'.

HEIGHT AND WEIGHT CENTILES MARKEDLY DISCREPANT

There is a marked or increasing discrepancy in the centile ranking between height and weight. Initially children will continue to grow in height and lose weight; it is only much later that height is affected. This discrepancy may also operate in reverse where there is increasing weight gain, leading to obesity, to the extent that the child's health is impaired.

ASSESSMENT AND MANAGEMENT

The process of assessing growth and managing failure to thrive has four interrelated stages:
- Measuring
- Recording and Monitoring
- Consultation and Referral
- Management

MEASURING INFANTS AND CHILDREN

Assessment of a child's growth is integral to any programme of child health promotion. The minimum level of weight monitoring in infancy is measurement at birth, at the six-week developmental check and at times of immunisation, that is at two, three and four months old. These weights facilitate the early detection of growth failure. Continue to make regular measurements if an abnormality in growth is suspected and plot them on the growth chart. Measure length and head circumference (in children less than two years old) if there is any doubt about the adequacy of the weight gain. Carefully follow the detailed instructions given on the charts on how to plot these measurements.

RECORDING AND MONITORING

Growth charts are essential in helping to identify normal and abnormal growth patterns. Routinely plot all measurements on the A5 growth charts within the Personal Child Health Record (PCHR). Babies are weighed naked; toddlers wear only pants. If abnormal weight and/or height loss or gain is found, ensure there are no calculation errors. If there are concerns about a child's growth, maintain parallel A4 charts in addition to the A5 chart in the PCHR. Keep these to facilitate monitoring and referral.

CONSULTATION AND REFERRAL

Discuss any perceived abnormal growth pattern with a more experienced colleague. Weight velocity changes significantly during the first two years of life, and many infants may cross up or down one or two centiles, particularly in the first year. A diagnosis of normal and adequate growth is very supportive for most parents; repeated weighing sometimes creates unnecessary anxiety, which itself is damaging.

Recognise and act on failure to thrive as early as possible, before patterns of poor nutrition and growth become entrenched. The condition can be difficult to acknowledge, lying as it does at the heart of what is considered to be 'good enough' parenting. There can be denial about it by both parents and professionals, and professional reluctance to discuss these issues with parents and refer promptly is potentially damaging for the child. Without active intervention children with failure to thrive may never reach their full potential.

MANAGEMENT
Once failure to thrive is identified, effective management includes addressing the underlying cause as well as taking steps to improve nutrition. In many cases where poor growth is the outcome of the wrong food or poor feeding techniques for example, it can be managed by the advice, support and monitoring from members of the primary health care team. However, if failure to thrive does not respond to this intervention then consider referral to the consultant paediatrician. When a diagnosis of non-organic failure to thrive is made, social services may need to become involved. View the management of non-organic failure to thrive as a multi-disciplinary and multi-agency responsibility. This will secure the best outcome for the child.

10

Abuse of children with disabilities

───────

CHILDREN WITH DISABILITIES can be and are abused. They are at a significantly higher risk of abuse than a child with no disability, while multiple disability compounds the possibility of both abuse and neglect. In our society disabled children tend to be treated differently from those who are non-disabled, often isolated physically, geographically and socially. They are more dependent on others for their care and more likely to spend time in residential care. Children with disabilities suffer abuse in all areas of life, whether in the home or at school, in foster or respite care, a hospital or hostel. Wherever it occurs abuse has the same damaging and long-term consequences for disabled children as it does for everyone else.

RELATIONSHIP BETWEEN DISABILITY AND ABUSE

Disabled children have a wide range of difficulties from the mild to the severe and the simple to the complex, which include physical, sensory (that is, hearing and vision) and/or learning difficulties. Children with learning difficulties comprise the largest single group of disabled children, and their problems will range from mild through moderate to severe. Many have multiple disabilities. In order to safeguard the disabled child it is important to appreciate both the nature and impact of a child's disability as well as the type of abuse and its effect on the child.

Abuse can be implicated in the cause of disability. Some children who have been physically abused (for example, severe shaking injury) may suffer permanent physical damage. Others with a history of abuse and neglect develop learning difficulties. The trauma of abuse potentially compounds a pre-existing disability and thereby increases the child's vulnerability.

The interrelationship between disability and abuse is complex. The maltreatment of children at home and in institutions covers a range of actions and behaviour, such as force feeding, segregation, discrimination, the use of physical restraints, confinement to a room or cot, over sedation or treatment without proper analgesia. Some methods used to treat children may be abusive in themselves. The lack of privacy of children with high dependency needs can be compounded by actions that may be perceived as abusive, such as opening letters, listening to telephone calls or public toileting.

WHAT MAKES CHILDREN WITH DISABILITIES MORE VULNERABLE TO ABUSE?

PREJUDICE AND STEREOTYPING
The prejudices and stereotypes that exist within our society about disability tend to make disabled children more vulnerable. They can be perceived negatively, as different and therefore inferior, either physically or cognitively. There may be more acceptance of the abuse than there is empathy for the child, a state of affairs reinforced by the following commonly held assumptions:

- Disabled children are unlikely to be abused because people feel sorry for them, and because they are not attractive
- Abuse (such as sexual abuse) would not be so harmful because disabled children would not understand it and would not feel it
- They would be more likely to make false allegations
- They would not benefit from therapy or treatment

POOR SELF-IMAGE

Many disabled children have low self-esteem. They may internalise a negative view of themselves and their disability, and believe, as a consequence, that they deserve the abuse. Their degree of disability can make it difficult for them to resist abuse (they may not be able to get away) or to disclose the maltreatment once it happens (they may not be able to communicate). Disabled children generally have fewer social contacts than other children, so they may not know who to tell, particularly if the perpetrator is a trusted adult who is also responsible for their care.

COMPLIANCE AND PASSIVITY

Compliance and passivity are qualities often fostered and rewarded in disabled children. Encouraged to do what they are told, they may therefore lack the confidence and assertiveness necessary to disclose abuse.

COMMUNICATION DIFFICULTIES

Children whose disability results in a lack of communication skills can find it difficult to express the experience of abuse and make it understood. Disabled children often do not have access to a means of communication.

LACK OF PHYSICAL BOUNDARIES

Age-appropriate physical boundaries do not exist for some disabled children, and it is often difficult for them to distinguish between touching that feels comfortable and appropriate, and touching that does not, particularly if most or all of their physical care is attended to by other people. The idea of 'private parts' has limited meaning for children who require help with basic toileting and dressing functions. Their isolation and inexperience may also mean that they are not necessarily aware of the limits of 'normal' behaviour.

NEED FOR LOVE AND AFFECTION

Disabled children may have experienced rejection and therefore limited opportunities for expressing and receiving love and affection.

Consequently, many have a desire to please and respond to the affection and closeness that often accompanies sexual abuse.

All the difficulties outlined above are compounded by the fact that the testimony of disabled children is less likely to be believed. Distressed by abuse and their desire for it to stop, their attempts to communicate may be misinterpreted as fantasy or challenging behaviour.

Many child safety programmes do not include the disabled child and their particular needs, and consequently disabled children receive less information on abuse and how to protect themselves from it. Safety strategies usually rely on a child's cognitive skills and ability to understand the difference between appropriate and inappropriate touch, something difficult for the disabled child.

A disabled child may be more immature, dependent, inexperienced, inarticulate and needy than a child without a disability. Remember perpetrators recognise their vulnerability, and they are aware of the difficulties that such children have not only in reporting abuse but also in being believed.

RECOGNISING ABUSE

The signs and indicators of abuse in children with any kind of disability can be confusing and wrongly attributed to the disability itself. Excessive masturbation and/or eroticised behaviour, for example, are often dismissed as expressions of an existing disability rather than a response to sexual abuse. This can be reinforced by adult reluctance to acknowledge that abuse may be taking place.

Working to safeguard children who have been abused or are at risk of abuse is a complex, stressful and demanding process, made harder when the child involved has a disability. In order to secure the best possible outcomes for disabled children always act upon concerns about their welfare in the very same way as for any other child.

11

Non-compliance

THERE WILL ALWAYS be parents/carers who do not wish to be helped by the professional network for a variety of reasons, and they have the right to exercise that choice. However, the refusal or reluctance of parents or carers to work in partnership with professionals where there are concerns about a child's welfare is known as non-compliance and should trigger further enquiries. Always consider whether non-compliance is concealing child abuse or neglect. The checklist below helps pinpoint those occasions when parental non-compliance could indicate that a child is at risk:

- Outright refusal of a service, such as child health promotion, with little explanation and/or refusal to allow the child to be seen
- Child has not been seen for long periods
- Covert refusal of service, for example arrangements are made but not kept, leading to repeated failed appointments at home and/or in clinic
- Failure to comply with appointments (such as, dentist, orthoptist, therapist, dietician, paediatric outpatients and so on) in circumstances that might jeopardise the child's health and development

Consider too the following:
- Hostile behaviour towards the health professional and/or other individuals
- Prior history of abuse and/or neglect of the child or sibling
- Current concerns about the child and capacity of parent to meet child's needs

- Families who have had a series of changes of address and children who change schools, nursery or general practitioner frequently
- Children who access accident and emergency departments rather than primary care

Parents sometimes withdraw from contact with the professional network when abuse is escalating. A professional may be regularly denied access to the home, the family may repeatedly fail to keep scheduled appointments and the child may stop attending nursery or school. In some circumstances a family may disappear altogether. If there is also a history of abuse the child may be at increased risk and vigilance is vital until there is evidence that the child is safe.

Equally parents may appear to comply and co-operate with professionals because they recognise that permitting limited access is a more effective way of keeping the professionals at bay than outright refusal. Some parents can be devious, manipulative and/or threatening. Many lie in order to conceal the abuse. Others evoke sympathy and demand the attention and support of the professional network in addressing their own needs. Whatever the circumstances, be suspicious if the apparent willingness of a parent to co-operate does not produce any change in the outcome for the child.

Judge each situation on its individual merits and in the context of all the available information about child and family. Inform other agencies and professionals who know the family. Refer to social services if there is any possibility that a parent's non-compliance is concealing abuse or neglect. When the parents/carers of a child who is on the child protection register do not comply with the child protection plan inform the key worker immediately with a view to reconvening a child protection conference.

12

The child protection conference

A CHILD PROTECTION CONFERENCE is a formal meeting convened by social services or the NSPCC. It is the principal forum for professionals and family to share information and concerns about a child seen to be at risk of continuing harm.

CHILD PROTECTION ENQUIRY AND INITIAL ASSESSMENT

The decision to initiate a child protection enquiry is made in a strategy meeting or discussion involving social services, police, health and other involved agencies. This will normally take place within one working day of a referral being received. All agencies involved with the child and family have a responsibility to share information at this stage so that a decision can be made about whether a child in need assessment or a child protection enquiry is needed. The aim of the enquiry process is to assess the child's needs and the capacity of the parents or wider family to ensure their safety and respond appropriately to their health and developmental needs. If a child is found to be at continuing risk of significant harm, a child protection conference is held.

THE CONFERENCE

The purpose of a child protection conference is to share information collected during the enquiry process, and to analyse and assess the degree of risk to an individual child or children within a family. Conference decides whether to place the child's name on the Child

Protection Register and makes recommendations for action in the form of a protection plan to safeguard the child and promote their welfare.

The conference includes parents and/or other carers and their representatives. Parents are encouraged to attend because in most cases they are key to the care and protection of their children. The Children Act 1989 places a duty of care on parents and a duty on the professional network to assist them in fulfilling their responsibility. Parents are rarely excluded from conferences. This only happens where their involvement may be thought to compromise the safety or well being of the child or otherwise interfere with the task of the conference to ensure the child's safety. The safety and welfare of the child is always the central and primary focus.

Conferences sometimes include children and their presence will depend on their age and level of understanding. In assessing a child's capacity to benefit from participating in the conference a balance needs to be struck between the child's need to be involved and yet to be protected from the stresses and conflicts of the process. Look at ways in which the child's views and feelings can be communicated to the conference irrespective of whether or not they are present.

The conference symbolises the multi-agency nature of the assessment and planning process. It draws together professionals from all agencies with specific responsibilities for the child and family (social services, health, police, education, probation and the voluntary sector) as well as others able to offer specialist advice (such as solicitors or housing officers). It provides a joint forum for conducting and agreeing a combined approach to work with the child and family to secure the best possible outcome for the child.

As part of this process health representation at conferences is vital and ensures that relevant details of the child's health, growth and development are known to all agencies involved in the protection of the child. Health professionals will also be able to give an opinion about the capacity of the parent/carer to keep the child from further harm and promote their health and development. The conference will not be able adequately to consider the risk to the child, nor make informed decisions and recommendations about their welfare, without a health professional present and/or their report.

The role of the child protection conference is to:

- Share relevant information about the child and family
- Assess risk to the child
- Decide about placement on the child protection register
- Appoint a key worker who must be a social worker or a nominee from the NSPCC
- Formulate the Child Protection Plan: the written plan of care specifies the expected changes and how they might reduce the risk of harm to the child over a certain time scale. It details each agency's contribution to the protection and welfare of the child and clarifies what is expected of the parents and what in turn the parents can expect of each agency. It identifies any further core and specialist assessments required
- Decide membership of the Core Group
- Agree about if and when to reconvene and review

There are two types of child protection conference: Initial and Review. The Initial Child Protection Conference is convened following a child protection enquiry. The subsequent use of the word 'Review' describes all the ensuing conferences. A Child Protection Review is held within four months of the initial conference and every six months thereafter until a decision is taken to remove the child's name from the child protection register. When there are concerns about the safety of an unborn child a Pre-Birth Child Protection Conference is held. Such conferences have the same status and are conducted in the same manner as Initial Child Protection Conferences.

CONFIDENTIALITY

Participants at child protection conferences are bound by the rules of confidentiality. They are expected to share information that is relevant to the protection of the child. Anything discussed at a conference is confidential to those participating and shared only on a strictly 'needs to know' basis, that is, with other professionals who hold responsibility for the protection of the child. Discuss any decision to withhold information that might adversely affect a child's safety and well being with either one of the designated or named professionals or other experienced colleague.

PREPARATION OF CONFERENCE REPORTS

Working Together to Safeguard Children states that all professionals attending a child protection conference should prepare a written report that may include growth charts if appropriate. The report should give an assessment of the child's health and development and any ongoing work that is relevant to the child's welfare. It should also provide information, where known, about relationships within the family that are pertinent to the protection of the child and any details that may highlight issues around the capacity of the parent/carer to meet the child's needs and promote their health and development.

All reports should distinguish between fact and observation, allegation and opinion, and support professional opinion with relevant evidence and/or research. Factual information should be clear, concise and relevant to the protection of the child. Make every effort not only to ensure that the parent is aware of the report's content but also to consider what the child needs to know in the context of their age and understanding.

The following checklist offers guidance to what might be included in the report. It does not provide an exhaustive list of risk factors. Nor can it indicate the nature, degree or severity of risk, which is a matter for individual professional judgement. Look at the relationship between a number of different factors. The fact that a child is not seen, for example, carries no risk in most cases. However, if this were to be combined with, say, a history of previous abuse, it might indicate a more serious concern.

FAMILY AND ENVIRONMENT

This includes factors that may influence a parent's/carer's capacity to respond appropriately to their child's needs and the impact of the wider family and social network. Examples might be: history of family violence and/or abuse, social isolation, unwanted pregnancy, substance misuse, mental health problems, families with diffuse social problems, housing, employment. A family genogram is helpful.

PARENTING CAPACITY

Remember to include the perceptions, views and feelings of parents and carers, and, where they are known, those of the child.

PHYSICAL CARE Assess the parents' capacity to meet child's physical needs and protect them from harm. Examples might include: lack of supervision, poor nutrition, poor hygiene, inadequate clothing, not meeting identified health needs, failed appointments, unsafe/chaotic home conditions with little or no evidence of provision of basic needs (food, warmth, adequate shelter, basic hygiene and toys)

EMOTIONAL/PSYCHOLOGICAL CARE Assess the parent–child relationship and the impact of any known relationship difficulties. Examples might include: unrealistic or developmentally inappropriate expectations, high criticism, little or no warmth, lack of understanding and responsiveness to child's needs, parental scapegoating or rejection of the child

THE CHILD

PHYSICAL HEALTH AND DEVELOPMENT Assess the child's appearance, growth and development. Make reference to growth charts, developmental checks, immunisation status, contacts with primary care team and other clinic/hospital attendance and their outcomes. Remember to include information on the child's past history.

EMOTIONAL AND PSYCHOLOGICAL HEALTH Assess the child's mood, non-verbal cues, behaviour, play, response to parent/siblings. Listen to what the child says and report any relevant allegation or disclosure. Identify and comment on behaviour that could indicate that the parent/carer's capacity to meet the child's needs is less than adequate. Examples might include: aggressive, attention-seeking behaviour, a withdrawn, wary, anxious or otherwise unhappy child, an over dependent child or inappropriate friendliness

Comment too on the protective factors for the child. Factors that may influence the outcome for the child include a secure attachment to the primary care giver, other non-abusive, secure and enduring relationships, and the opportunity to excel in their own right, e.g. achievement at school

FAMILY STRENGTHS/PROTECTIVE FACTORS
Include elements within the family with the potential to minimise risk to the child, the strong and positive aspects of the parent–child relationship as well as its weak and negative side. This creates a balanced view of the parent/carer's capacity to provide adequate care and their potential to make whatever changes necessary to meet this need in the future. Examples of protective factors in families might include a parent with insight into the problem, one prepared to take appropriate responsibility and accept the need to work with the professionals to achieve change. Or the existence of an involved extended family network willing to assume some responsibility for the child's welfare and support the parents in providing good-enough care. Or family difficulties where the child is not blamed and the parent can see the world from their point of view.

ASSESSMENT OF RISK
Look at the relationship between the evidence of ill treatment or lack of care and its impact on the child in order to reach a view about the risk of significant harm to the child. Focus perhaps on one particular issue seen to have overriding significance, or summarise the principal issues identified in some or all of the previous four sections.

FUTURE PLAN OF WORK
Clarify the role and contribution of each service in meeting the needs of the child and family. Revise this perhaps after the conference when the multi-agency assessment, decision-making and planning process is complete.

THE CHILD PROTECTION REGISTER
The conference decides whether or not to place the child on the child protection register. In making this decision it should consider the following question:

- **Is the child at continuing risk of significant harm?**

The test should be that either:

■ the child can be shown to have suffered ill-treatment or impairment of health or development as a result of physical, emotional or sexual abuse, or neglect, and professional judgement is that further ill-treatment or impairment is likely; or
■ professional judgement, substantiated by the findings of enquiries in this individual case or by research evidence, is that the child is likely to suffer ill-treatment or the impairment of health or development as a result of physical, emotional, or sexual abuse or neglect

Working Together to Safeguard Children (DH, 1999)

The conference needs to establish, as far as possible, the cause of harm or the likelihood of harm. This is something that might apply to siblings or other children in the same household and justify their assessment and subsequent registration too. Children are categorised according to the area of concern and the chair of the conference will decide under which category or categories of abuse the child's name is registered.

Express any disagreement with the majority view and ensure any dissent and the reason for it is recorded in the minutes. Issues arising from a lack of consensus at a conference may require further discussion if the dissenter wishes to challenge the decision reached by the conference. Discuss this with one of the named or designated professionals or other experienced colleague.

The act of registration does not in itself confer protection on a child, and the accompanying protection plan should specify what needs to change to ensure that the child is protected from harm in the future. The purpose of the register, which is held by social services, is to:

■ Alert professionals to the need for continued surveillance
■ Indicate to those consulting the register the primary concern at the time of registration
■ Provide a source of data for looking at trends in child abuse and neglect

The child protection register is not a record of all children who have been abused. It contains the names of children about whom there are unresolved child protection issues and for whom there is an inter-agency protection plan.

CORE ASSESSMENT

All children placed on the child protection register are subject to a core assessment that builds on the information already gathered during the enquiry process, initial assessment and conference. This has to be done in accordance with the child protection plan and comply with the guidance in the *Framework for the Assessment of Children in Need and their Families*. The assessment framework is represented in the form of a pyramid with the child's welfare at the centre (see Appendix 1). Its core dimensions are the child's developmental needs, the parent's capacity to respond appropriately to those needs and the impact of wider family and environmental factors. An assessment integrating these three systems or 'domains' provides the basis for understanding what is happening to a child and has been developed to provide a framework that is common to all agencies. Health professionals will be expected to contribute to the core assessment and to provide or arrange specialist assessments where appropriate.

CORE GROUPS

Inter-agency Core Group meetings take place between conferences. They involve the parent/carer, key worker and any professional within the multi-agency network directly involved in the implementation of the child protection plan. In some cases the child is also involved. Their function is to undertake the assessment, co-ordinate and develop the work agreed upon in the child protection plan and monitor its progress in the light of any objectives set at the conference.

13

Records

PROFESSIONAL ACCOUNTABILITY IS made formal and explicit through the accurate recording of information. This is an essential prerequisite for effective communication and as such plays a crucial part in safeguarding children.

BASIC PRINCIPLES

Written communication in the form of good record keeping and effective verbal communication go hand in hand. Good documentation can shape the view of a case, clarify objectives, stimulate further action and in this way form the basis for sound professional decision-making. Where there is concern about the safety and welfare of a child, ensure that this is accurately reflected in the child's records. Include a precise and detailed account of the event/contact, the decision reached and any action plan and/or referral. Include discussions with other professionals. Distinguish between what is observation, suspicion and opinion.

The record should be contemporaneous with the contact or otherwise written within 24 hours of it. In all cases note the date and place of contact and remember to sign it. Check that the current and previous names of the child, the address, date of birth, GP and current day care/nursery/school are recorded. Include the names of all adults who have parental responsibility and/or who live with the child; concerns about any of this information should trigger further enquiries.

The record should be legible, continuous and clear; the information systematically stored and easy to access. It is for other professionals to read as well; they should be able to find historical information easily and use what is already known about the child and family in the ongoing assessment and planning process. Ensure there is a mechanism to highlight those children about whom there are child protection concerns, for both written and computer records.

Once a child is known to have moved, ensure that primary care records follow them as speedily as possible. Send letters and discharge summaries promptly with copies to professionals and parents as appropriate. This will enable historical information from a number of sources to be integrated into current assessments.

Tell parents/carers and children about their health records. One of the principles of 'working in partnership' is that parents and children (depending on their age and understanding) are kept informed of what is recorded and why. Explain too why information needs to be shared with others. Involve them by completing the record with them and give them copies where appropriate. Remember all records are legal documents and can be used as evidence in legal proceedings as well as being read by the parent and sometimes the child. In addition parents may also have access to copies of correspondence that are held by a third party, for example social services.

CONFIDENTIALITY AND INFORMATION SHARING

The sharing of information should operate in accordance with the Data Protection Act 1998, and all health service trusts now have a responsibility for improving the way that the NHS handles and protects patient information. The general principles of the Act are that:

- **There is a general common law duty to safeguard the confidentiality of personal information**
- **Decisions to disclose information or to refuse a request for disclosure from another agency or individual should always be clearly recorded**

However, the degree of confidentiality should always be governed by the need to protect the child. Under certain circumstances the Act does allow for the disclosure of information without the consent of the individual concerned. Discuss disclosure of all or part of any record with the parent and/or child (depending on their age and understanding), and seek and obtain their consent where possible. If agreement is withheld, and there is professional concern about the risk of harm to a child, disclose any relevant information. Make any disclosure on a strictly 'needs to know' basis, that is to other professionals who share responsibility for protecting the child.

Ensure that maintaining the confidentiality of the record does not become a barrier to communication that places a child at further risk. If in doubt and concerned that withholding information may adversely affect a child's safety and well being, discuss with one of the named or designated professionals or other experienced colleague.

CALDICOTT STANDARDS

The Caldicott standards are based on the principles of the Data Protection Act; they provide a framework for the management of confidentiality and access to personal information for the NHS and social services. This includes standards for the secure storage and transfer of confidential information/records and local arrangements for information sharing within health and social services have to comply with these standards. However, they do not prevent the sharing of information where there are concerns about the safety and welfare of a child.

14

The legal framework

THE CHILDREN ACT 1989 sets out the legal requirements for child protection practice. The Act introduces orders applicable when children are at risk of significant harm. Public and private laws relating to children are combined under it, in a series of principles governing practice and procedure, both in and out of court.

MAIN PRINCIPLES OF THE CHILDREN ACT 1989

- Welfare of the child is paramount
- Children should be brought up and cared for within their own families, wherever possible
- Children in danger should be kept safe and protected by effective intervention
- Agencies should work in partnership with parents insofar as this does not prejudice the welfare of the child
- Delays in decisions affecting children are likely to prejudice their welfare. Courts should ensure that delay is avoided and make an order only if to do so is better than not
- Children should be informed about what is happening to them, and their wishes and feelings taken into account (considered in the light of their age and understanding). They should have the opportunity to participate in decisions being made about their future
- Parents continue to have parental responsibility in relation to their children, even if their children are no longer living with them. They should be kept informed about their children and participate in decisions made about their future

- Parents with children in need should be helped to bring them up themselves
- Help should be provided as a service to the child and their family and:
    - Be provided in partnership with the parents
    - Meet each child's identified needs
    - Be appropriate to the child's race, culture, religion and language
    - Be open to effective, independent representations and complaints procedures
    - Draw upon effective partnership between the local authority and other agencies, including voluntary agencies

PARENTAL RESPONSIBILITY

Responsibility is the key word here. Although defined as all the rights, duties, powers, responsibilities and authority that by law the parent of a child has in relation to that child, the legal emphasis is on responsibility. Parents are expected to be responsible for looking after their children, and local authorities have a duty to support them in so doing as the need arises.

Parental responsibility may be shared by a number of people. The birth mother always has parental responsibility (unless it has been lost through the child being adopted). The birth father has parental responsibility jointly with the mother only if they marry at any time before or after the child's conception. Parental responsibility can be acquired by other adults, such as the unmarried father, grandparents or step-parents, through a Parental Responsibility Order. The local authority can also acquire parental responsibility through the making of a Care Order. If parental responsibility is acquired through a court order, such as a Residence Order, it will be lost when the order ends.

Establish who has parental responsibility when seeking consent for treatment, for example immunisation.

SIGNIFICANT HARM AND COURT PROCEDURES

The sole ground for initiating proceedings under the Children Act 1989 is that the child is suffering or is likely to suffer significant harm, and that the harm, or likelihood of harm, is attributable to:

- Care given to the child, or likely to be given to them, if the order were not made, not being what it would be reasonable to expect a parent to give to them, or
- The child being beyond parental control

In reaching a decision about a child the court considers:

- The comparison of the child's health and development with a similar child
- Whether the care given by the parents should be what might reasonably be expected
- Whether minor shortcomings in care or deficits in development may have a cumulative effect and result in significant harm

The court's Welfare Checklist therefore includes the following:

- Wishes of the child
- Child's physical, emotional and educational needs
- Likely effect of any change in their circumstances
- Age, sex, cultural background and any other characteristic the court considers relevant
- Any harm the child has suffered or is at risk of suffering
- Capability of the child's parents or any other potential carer to provide reasonable parental care

In some applications for court orders, primarily care applications, the court appoints a children's guardian (formerly guardian *ad litem*), someone who reports on and makes recommendations about the child to the court. Guardians are independent practitioners, usually social workers, who are responsible for helping the court reach a decision about a child. The guardian is entitled to inspect social services files and to request information or copies of documents relating to the child from any other agency involved. The children's guardian does not have right of access to the child's medical notes. Authority to see these records must be sought from whomever has parental responsibility.

CONFIDENTIALITY

All health service workers are expected to maintain the confidentiality of patient/client information and all professional regulatory bodies have their own code of conduct in relation to this. However, the willingness of professionals to share confidential information is crucial where there are concerns about the safety or well being of a child.

In child protection practice there are three ways in which the disclosure of confidential information can be justified:

- **With the consent of the parent/carer and/or child**
- **Without consent when the disclosure is required by law or by order of the court**
- **Without consent when disclosure is considered necessary in the public interest. This includes child abuse**

The issue of consent is one that presents most difficulty for health care workers. There will be occasions where abuse or neglect is suspected and it is either not possible to gain consent for information to be disclosed or consent is actively withheld. The person withholding consent may be the victim, the perpetrator of the abuse or another person. Whatever the circumstances, the primary duty and responsibility of the professional is to act in the child's best interests. Although disclosure without consent should be the exception rather than the rule, it is lawful to disclose confidential information if it appears necessary to do so to safeguard a child in the 'public interest'. What this means in practice is that the public interest in protecting children may override the public interest in maintaining confidentiality. Remember to disclose information that is relevant to the concern about the child and to share information on a 'needs to know' basis, that is with other professionals who have a duty of care towards the child.

GILLICK (NOW KNOWN AS THE FRASER RULING)

The Gillick case concerned the right of a young person under 16 years of age to consent for medical treatment without the parents' knowledge. The subsequent ruling said that a young person can be considered competent to consent to treatment if their age and understanding are sufficient to enable them to understand what is involved. The concept of competence is central to the law's approach to consent. The Fraser ruling defines competence as an ability to understand information about a proposed treatment. However, in practice it may be difficult to define the level of understanding required for a particular treatment or procedure. There is no easy test of competence for young people and the ability to understand may not necessarily be the same as actual understanding. If in doubt about the capacity of a child to consent, consult one of the named or designated professionals or other experienced colleague.

The assessment framework

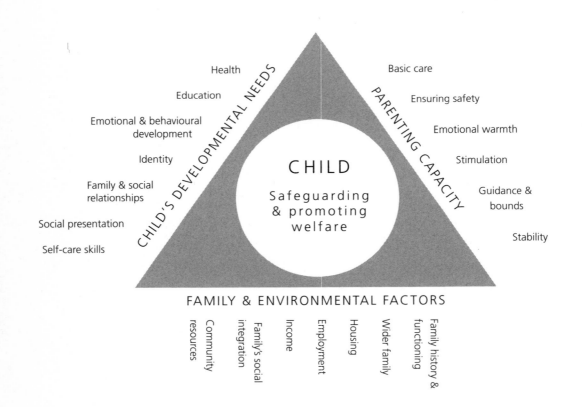

CHILD'S DEVELOPMENTAL NEEDS

Health

Education

Emotional & behavioural development

Identity

Family & social relationships

Social presentation

Self-care skills

PARENTING CAPACITY

Basic care

Ensuring safety

Emotional warmth

Stimulation

Guidance & bounds

Stability

CHILD

Safeguarding & promoting welfare

FAMILY & ENVIRONMENTAL FACTORS

Community resources

Family's social integration

Income

Employment

Housing

Wider family

Family history & functioning

Dimensions of child's developmental needs

HEALTH
Includes growth and development as well as physical and mental well being. The impact of genetic factors and of any impairment need to be considered. Involves receiving appropriate health care when ill, an adequate and nutritious diet, exercise, immunisations where appropriate and developmental checks, dental and optical care and, for older children, appropriate advice and information on issues that have an impact on health, including sex education and substance misuse.

EDUCATION
Covers all areas of a child's cognitive development, which begins from birth. Includes opportunities: for play and interaction with other children to have access to books; to acquire a range of skills and interests; to experience success and achievement. Involves an adult interested in educational activities, progress and achievements, who takes account of the child's starting point and any special educational needs.

EMOTIONAL AND BEHAVIOURAL DEVELOPMENT
Concerns the appropriateness of response demonstrated in feelings and actions by a child, initially to parents and caregivers and, as the child grows older, to others beyond the family. Includes nature and quality of early attachments, characteristics of temperament, adaptation to change, response to stress and degree of appropriate self control.

IDENTITY
Concerns the child's growing sense of self as a separate and valued person. Includes the child's view of self and abilities, self image and self esteem, and having a positive sense of individuality. Race religion, age, gender, sexuality and disability may all contribute to this. Feelings of belonging and acceptance by family, peer group and wider society, including other cultural groups.

FAMILY AND SOCIAL RELATIONSHIPS

Development of empathy and the capacity to place self in someone else's shoes. Includes a stable and affectionate relationship with parents or caregivers, good relationships with siblings, increasing importance of age appropriate friendships with peers and other significant persons in the child's life and response of family to these relationships.

SOCIAL PRESENTATION

Concerns child's growing understanding of the way in which appearance, behaviour, and any impairment are perceived by the outside world and the impression being created. Includes appropriateness of dress for age, gender, culture and religion; cleanliness and personal hygiene; and availability of advice from parents or caregivers about presentation in different settings.

SELF-CARE SKILLS

Concerns the acquisition by a child of practical, emotional and communication competencies required for increasing independence. Includes early practical skills of dressing and feeding, opportunities to gain confidence and practical skills to undertake activities away from the family and independent living skills as older children. Includes encouragement to acquire social problem solving approaches. Special attention should be given to the impact of a child's impairment and other vulnerabilities, and on social circumstances affecting these in the development of self-care skills.

Dimensions of parenting capacity

BASIC CARE
Providing for the child's physical needs, and appropriate medical and dental care.

- Includes provision of food, drink, warmth, shelter, clean and appropriate clothing and adequate personal hygiene.

ENSURING SAFETY
Ensuring the child is adequately protected from harm or danger.

- Includes protection from significant harm or danger, and from contact with unsafe adults/other children and from self-harm. Recognition of hazards and danger both in the home and elsewhere.

EMOTIONAL WARMTH
Ensuring the child's emotional needs are met, giving the child a sense of being specially valued and a positive sense of own racial and cultural identity.

- Includes ensuring the child's requirements for secure, stable and affectionate relationships with significant adults, with appropriate sensitivity and responsiveness to the child's needs. Appropriate physical contact, comfort and cuddling sufficient to demonstrate warm regard, praise and encouragement.

STIMULATION
Promoting child's learning and intellectual development through encouragement and cognitive stimulation and promoting social opportunities.

- Includes facilitating the child's cognitive development and potential through interaction, communication, talking and responding to the child's language and questions, encouraging and joining the child's play, and promoting educational opportunities. Enabling the child to experience success and ensuring school attendance or equivalent opportunity. Facilitating child to meet challenges of life.

GUIDANCE AND BOUNDARIES
Enabling the child to regulate their own emotions and behaviour.

The key parental tasks are demonstrating and modelling appropriate behaviour and control of emotions and interactions with others, and guidance that involves setting boundaries, so that the child is able to develop an internal model of moral values and conscience, and social behaviour appropriate for the society within which they will grow up. The aim is to enable the child to grow into an autonomous adult, holding their own values, and able to demonstrate appropriate behaviour with others rather than having to be dependent on rules outside themselves. This includes not over protecting children from exploratory and learning experiences.

■ Includes social problem solving, anger management, consideration for others, and effective discipline and shaping of behaviour.

STABILITY
Providing a sufficiently stable family environment to enable a child to develop and maintain a secure attachment to the primary caregiver(s) in order to ensure optimal development. Includes: ensuring secure attachments are not disrupted, providing consistency of emotional warmth over time and responding in a similar manner to the same behaviour. Parental responses change and develop according to child's developmental progress. In addition, ensuring children keep in contact with important family members and significant others.

Family and environmental factors

FAMILY HISTORY AND FUNCTIONING
Family history includes both genetic and psycho-social factors.

Family functioning is influenced by who is living in the household and how they are related to the child; significant changes in family/household composition; history of childhood experiences of parents; chronology of significant life events and their meaning to family members; nature of family functioning, including sibling relationships and its impact on the child; parental strengths and difficulties, including those of an absent parent; the relationship between separated parents.

WIDER FAMILY
Who are considered to be members of the wider family by the child and the parents? This includes related and non-related persons and absent wider family. What is their role and importance to the child and parents and in precisely what way?

HOUSING
Does the accommodation have basic amenities and facilities appropriate to the age and development of the child and other resident members? Is the housing accessible and suitable to the needs of disabled family members? Includes the interior and exterior of the accommodation and immediate surroundings. Basic amenities include water, heating, sanitation, cooking facilities, sleeping arrangements and cleanliness, hygiene and safety and their impact on the child's upbringing.

EMPLOYMENT
Who is working in the household, their pattern of work and any changes? What impact does this have on the child? How is work or absence of work viewed by family members? How does it affect their relationship with the child? Includes children's experience of work and its impact on them.

INCOME
Income available over a sustained period of time. Is the family in receipt of all its benefit entitlements? Sufficiency of income to meet the family's needs. The way resources available to the family are used. Are there financial difficulties that affect the child?

FAMILY'S SOCIAL INTEGRATION
Exploration of the wider context of the local neighbourhood and community and its impact on the child and parents. Includes the degree of the family's integration or isolation, their peer groups, friendship and social networks and the importance attached to them.

COMMUNITY RESOURCES
Describes all facilities and services in a neighbourhood, including universal services of primary health care, day care and schools, places of worship, transport, shops and leisure activities. Includes availability, accessibility and standard of resources and impact on the family, including disabled members.

The paediatric assessment

Where there is actual or suspected child abuse and/or neglect, a paediatric assessment may be essential as it can provide an independent opinion that is helpful for professionals, parents and the child. Approach the assessment of the child in a rigorous and systematic way irrespective of whether there is an allegation of abuse, unexplained injury or the incidental discovery of abuse and/or neglect. The diagnostic process does not differ from the diagnostic process in any other disorder although it will occur within a multi-agency context of assessment and planning for the child.

Document findings fully; make clear, precise and contemporaneous notes and sign them. Use body maps wherever possible or draw diagrams, label and sign. Distinguish between the history, observations, suspicions and interpretations. List the necessary investigations and referrals. The consultant for the child should validate a trainee's notes.

HISTORY

Take a full paediatric history that includes:

- **Views and feelings of the child**
- **Name of the person giving the history and relationship to child**
- **Duration and frequency of the alleged abuse**
- **Time and date of first episode**
- **Time and date of last episode**
- **Other injuries, e.g. genital, old injuries**

- Past history
- Developmental history and immunisation status
- Behavioural and emotional problems including symptoms of post-traumatic stress
- Social history including current members of household and child-care arrangements
- Siblings, safety and wellbeing
- Family history, genogram
- Family networks and other carers

Remember, in cases involving a memorandum interview work closely with the police to avoid unnecessary history taking and /or contamination of evidence.

EXAMINATION

Remember, in relation to the examination, to do the following:

- Ask the child for permission
- Try and allow the child some control of the situation and respect their wishes
- Talk to the child before and during the examination
- Explain the process: respect privacy and build up the child's confidence
- Allow the child to choose who they want to be with during the examination
- Examine genitalia and anus at end of the examination
- Never use physical restraint (pre-verbal infants need to be held by their parent/carer)
- Evaluate demeanour, response to carer, play, attention, behaviour during the examination
- Record whether or not the child was able to co-operate. If the examination is incomplete, record explanation of how and why
- Measure height, weight and head circumference. Record and plot the centiles

- Conduct a thorough general physical examination to include hair, nails, mouth, ears, nose, head and fundi.
- Examine the cardiovascular, respiratory, abdominal and central nervous systems
- Comment on development. Conduct a brief examination if appropriate or recommend a follow-up appointment to assess development
- Note the pubertal stage
- Take photographs if appropriate

Separate old injuries from new injuries and document the following:
- Site
- Size: measure and draw on body charts
- Colour
- Stage of healing
- Explanation of each injury as given by child and/or parent
- Bruises: describe your findings and note colour. (The only reliable dating of a bruise is that yellow indicates injury older than 24 hours)

Examination of genitalia and anus If during the course of taking the history and doing the examination sexual abuse is suspected, consider a detailed examination of the genitalia and anus. This is indicated when, for example, there is genital bleeding or disclosure of sexual abuse; in some cases forensic samples may be required. Guidance from the Royal College of Paediatrics and Child Health (2002) outlines the competencies needed for a single or joint examination and recommends photo documentation via a colposcope.

GENITALIA
- *In Boys* Look for injury to the urethra, penis and scrotum, such as bruises, tears, lacerations and burns. Always comment on the position of the testes and whether or not the child is circumcised
- *In Girls* Note any injuries to the external genitalia. Remember to include the lower abdomen and upper thighs. Examine the vulval area for abrasions, lacerations or discharge. With labial traction

describe the hymenal opening, dimensions, mobility, margin, presence of notches, bumps, tears and scars. Comment on the urethra, vestibule, vagina and posterior fourchette. Examine young girls on their mother's knee; older girls can lie supine on the couch in a 'frog-leg' position. Use a good light and, if available, a colposcope.

ANUS
- Examine in the left lateral position
- Buttocks must be separated for 30 seconds to observe the anal sphincters, look for reflex anal dilation (RAD)
- Note the extent of any injury, e.g. bruising, reddening or swelling of the skin and perineum
- Look at the anal margin
- Comment on ruggae
- Look for fissures/scars and describe their position, length and stage of healing

DIAGNOSIS/OPINION
- Give an opinion on whether the findings are consistent with the history given
- Decide whether the findings indicate accidental injury or non-accidental injury and abuse and/or neglect
- If there is uncertainty and/or no diagnosis, say so and outline next steps – i.e. investigations, further referrals, etc.
- Comment on other findings from history and examination, such as growth or language development

MANAGEMENT
- Arrange investigations to exclude an ascertainable causes
- Consider the immediate support available to the family
- Consider whether siblings are at risk
- Inform the Primary Care Team of the outcome of the assessment
- Consider referrals to other professionals, e.g. child and family consultation service, adult mental health services
- Obtain past records and complete a medical chronology reassessing current findings in the light of the past history

Paediatric follow-up may be necessary in certain cases in order to:
- Further assess symptoms and signs
- Find evidence of healing and/or of further abuse
- Diagnose underlying medical disorders or other co-existing conditions e.g. screening for sexually transmitted infections
- Provide a further detailed developmental assessment if appropriate

Remember
- Paediatric assessment is only part of the jigsaw that makes up the whole picture
- Discuss findings with the child, parents, social worker and police as appropriate; being suspicious of a parent and knowing when and how to express your concerns may be difficult; discuss with a senior doctor/consultant
- Parents, police and social services often want an instant opinion in a situation where there may be uncertainty and/or no diagnosis; in such cases always explain the differential diagnosis
- Submit typed statements for the police; consider seeking advice of senior colleague.

CONFIDENTIALITY

The General Medical Council guidelines in *Standards of Practice: Protecting and Providing Information* (2000) reiterates the importance of obtaining a patient's consent to the disclosure of information. It also makes it clear that personal information may be released without consent to third parties in exceptional circumstances, e.g. agencies such as social services or the police:

'If you believe a patient to be a victim of neglect or physical, sexual or emotional abuse and that the patient cannot give or withhold consent to disclosure, you should give information promptly to an appropriate responsible person or statutory agency, where you believe that the disclosure is in the patient's best interests. You should usually inform the patient that you intend to disclose the information before doing so. Such circumstances may arise in relation to children, where concerns about possible abuse need to be shared with other agencies such as social services. Where appropriate you should inform those with parental responsibility about the disclosure. If, for any reason, you believe that disclosure of information is not in the best interests of an abused or neglected patient, you must still be prepared to justify your decision'.

The GMC also confirms that its guidance refers to information about adults who may pose a risk to children as well as children who may be victims of abuse.

CONSENT

The child's consent is necessary for a medical or psychiatric examination if he or she has sufficient understanding to make an informed decision. Examination without consent may be held in law to be an assault. When assessing a child's capacity to decide whether to give or refuse consent, consider the following laws or legal precedents:

- At age 16 a young person can be treated as an adult and can be presumed to have capacity to decide
- Under age 16 children may have capacity to decide (Gillick ruling), depending on their ability to understand what is involved
- Where a competent child refuses treatment, a person with parental responsibility or the court may authorise medical or psychiatric examinations or treatment if this is considered to be in the child's best interests

When thinking about a child's capacity to consent, consider his or her:

- Ability to understand that there is a choice and that choices have consequences
- Willingness and ability to make a choice, including the option of choosing that someone else makes it
- Understanding of the nature and purpose of the proposed procedure, including the risks and benefits

Investigation of suspected non-accidental injury

Investigate any presenting symptoms or signs that appear to be suspicious and possibly result from non-accidental injury. Discuss individual cases with a senior doctor/consultant as necessary.

ABDOMINAL INJURY

Confirm the presence and site of a perforation and other abdominal injury with a surgical opinion.

BLOOD

- Serial haematocrit for blood loss
- Serum amylase (pancreatic and in some cases of splenic injury)
- Serum aspartate aminotransferase, alanine aminotransferase, lactate dehydrogenase (raised in liver injury)

URINE

- Gross or microscopic haematuria (greater than 20 red blood cells per high power field suggests damage to kidney or urinary tract)

RADIOLOGY

- Chest X-ray: rib fracture, pneumothorax and pleural fluid/haemothorax
- Postero-anterior abdominal and chest radiographs: supine and erect. Looking for free air and fluid levels
- Plain X-rays of abdomen: ground glass, intraperitoneal haemorrhage
- CT scanning: injury to lungs, pleura, solid abdominal organs, including pancreatic injury and duodenal haematoma

BONY INJURY

X-RAY

Refer for an x-ray as appropriate and in particular when there is localised pain, limp or reluctance to use a limb

SKELETAL SURVEY
Refer for a skeletal survey when a child dies in suspicious or unusual circumstances and consider it for:
- Physically abused children under 3 years
- Unexplained neurological symptoms or signs
- Where there is a fracture suggesting abuse
- Past history of suspicious skeletal injury
- Older children with severe soft-tissue injury

Remember to follow the local guidelines for a skeletal survey

DIFFERENTIAL DIAGNOSIS OF BONY INJURY
Consider the following laboratory tests
- Blood culture, white blood count – osteomyelitis
- Calcium, phosphate, alkaline phosphatase – rickets
- X-ray wrist and skull – osteogenesis imperfecta
- Serum copper, full blood count, caeruloplasmin – copper deficiency (rare)

BRUISING, BLEEDING OR PURPURA

FIRST-LINE INVESTIGATIONS
- Full blood count, platelet count and film (reviewed by Consultant Haematologist)
- Coagulation screen:
  - Prothrombin time (PT)
  - Activated partial thromboplastin time (APTT)
  - Thrombin time
  - Fibrinogen

Platelet function defect is not excluded by these tests. If suspected, discuss with a haematologist and take a drug history (salicylates, for example, can induce a platelet disorder).

SECOND-LINE INVESTIGATIONS
- Von Willebrand screen
- Factor assays
- Platelet aggregation studies
- Bleeding time

SHAKEN BABY/SUBDURAL HAEMATOMA/SUSPECTED HEAD INJURY

Consider the following investigations when serious abuse is suspected, or signs or symptoms indicate the possibility of intracranial injury:
- Skeletal survey (includes skull X-ray)
- CT scan of head (ultrasound also used) to identify acute trauma
- Skilled examination of eyes and optic fundi by an ophthalmologist
- Full blood count and serial haematocrit to detect further bleeding
- Clotting studies to exclude rare causes of bleeding
- Lumbar puncture/subdural tap: blood/xanthochromia

SUDDEN UNEXPLAINED DEATH

Investigate to exclude ascertainable causes. Sudden Infant Death Syndrome (SIDS) confirmed at post-mortem needs to be distinguished from fatal child abuse. During resuscitation take samples for:
- Toxicology
- Inherited metabolic diseases
- Cultures – bacterial and viral
- Chromosomes

Consider skin, liver and muscle biopsies. Undertake a skeletal survey if there are suspicions of physical abuse.

Suggested reading

Adcock M, White R (eds) (1998) *Significant Harm*, Significant Publications.

Amiel S, Heath I (eds) (2003) *Family Violence in Primary Care,* Oxford University Press.

The Bridge Child Care Consultancy Service (1995) *Paul, Death through Neglect*, Islington Area Child Protection Committee.

Browne K, Davies C, Stratton P M (eds) (2002) *Early Prediction and Prevention of Child Abuse*, Wiley.

Cawson P, Wattam C, Brooker S, Kelly G (2000) *Child Maltreatment in the United Kingdom: A Study of the Prevalence of Child Abuse and Neglect*, NSPCC.

Department of Health (1995) *Child Protection: Messages from Research*, HMSO.

Department of Health (1999) *Working Together to Safeguard Children*, The Stationery Office.

Department of Health (2000) *Framework for the Assessment of Children In Need and their Families*, The Stationery Office.

Department of Health (2000) *Safeguarding Children Involved in Prostitution: Supplementary Guidance to Working Together to Safeguard Children*, The Stationery Office.

Department of Health (2002) *Learning from Past Experience – A Review of Serious Case Reviews*, The Stationery Office.

Department of Health (2002) *Safeguarding Children in whom Illness is Induced or Fabricated by Carers with Parenting Responsibilities*, The Stationery Office.

Department of Health (2002) *Safeguarding Children – A Joint Chief Inspectors' Report on Arrangements to Safeguard Children*, The Stationery Office.

Department of Health (2003) *What to Do If You're Worried a Child is Being Abused: Children's Services Guidance,* The Stationery Office.

Gopfert M, Webster J and Seeman M V (eds) (2003) *Parental Psychiatric Disorder: Distressed Parents and their Families*, Cambridge University Press.

Heger A H, Emans S J, Muram M D (2000) *Evaluation of the Sexually Abused Child*, Oxford University Press.

Hobbs C J, Hanks H, Wynne J M (1999) *Child Abuse and Neglect: A Clinician's Handbook*, Churchill Livingstone.

Hobbs C J, Wynne J M (2001) *Physical Signs of Child Abuse: A Colour Atlas*, W B Saunders.

Howarth J (2001) *The Child's World*, Jessica Kingsley.

Iwaniec D (1995) *The Emotionally Abused and Neglected Child*, Wiley.

Jones D P H, Ramchandanl P (1999) *Child Sexual Abuse: Informing Practice from Research*, Radcliffe Medical Press.

Lord Laming *The Victoria Climbié Inquiry* (2003) The Stationery Office.

May-Chahal C, Coleman S (2003) *Safeguarding Children and Young People*, Routledge.

Meadow R (ed.) (1997) *ABC of Child Abuse*, 3rd edn, BMJ Books.

Mullender A, Morley R (eds) (1994) *Children Living with Domestic Violence*, Whiting & Birch.

Parton N (ed.) (1997) *Child Protection and Family Support: Tensions, Contradictions and Possibilities*, Routledge.

Reder P, Duncan S (1999) *Lost Innocents: A Follow-up Study of Fatal Child Abuse*, Routledge.

Reder P, Duncan S, Gray M (1993) *Beyond Blame: Child Abuse Tragedies Revisited*, Routledge.

Reder P, Lucey C (1995) *Assessment of Parenting: Psychiatric and Psychological Perspectives*, Routledge.

Rogers S, Hevey D, Ash E (1989) *Child Abuse and Neglect: An Introduction*, Open University.

Royal College of Paediatrics and Child Health (2002) *Fabricated or Induced Illness by Carers*, Royal College of Paediatrics and Child Health.

Royal College of Paediatrics and Child Health and the Association of Police Surgeons (2002) *Guidance on Paediatric Forensic Examinations in Relation to Possible Child Sexual Abuse*.

Royal College of Physicians of London (1997) *Physical Signs of Sexual Abuse in Children*, RCP Publications.

Ryan M (2000) *Working with Fathers*, Radcliffe Medical Press.

Stevenson O (1998) *Child Welfare in the UK*, Blackwell.

Stevenson O, Thompson P (1998) *Neglected Children: Issues and Dilemmas*, Blackwell.

Index